Respiratory
Facts

Respiratory Facts

John H. Riggs, B.A., R.R.T.
Respiratory Care Education and
Clinical Coordinator of ICN
Wake Medical Center
Raleigh, North Carolina
(Formerly, Director of Clinical Education
University of Charleston)

F. A. DAVIS COMPANY • Philadelphia

Printed in the United States of America

Last digit indicates print number: 10 9 8 7 6 5 4 3 2 1

Library of Congress Cataloging-in-Publication Data

Riggs, John, 1955–
   Respiratory facts.

   Includes bibliographies and index.
   1. Respiratory therapy — Handbooks, manuals, etc.
I. Title.
RC735.I5R54   1989   615.8'36   88-20257
ISBN 0-8036-7333-7

To Susan and Danielle

To:

York High School
Yorktown, Virginia

The University of Charleston
College of Health Science
Charleston, West Virginia

In Memory of Ed Clairmont, M.M.Sc., R.R.T.

Preface

Respiratory Facts is intended for respiratory care practitioners and respiratory therapy technology students who require a clear, concise, yet comprehensive guide to respiratory care facts and procedures. This guide is designed to be equally usable in hospital as well as home health care settings. For optimal utilization of this guide, a basic understanding of anatomy, physiology, and basic health care procedures is presupposed.

Respiratory Facts is written in a succinct style that offers the reader the maximum of information with the minimum of words. All explanations are clearly written and are reinforced with carefully formatted tables, charts, and graphs. Recognizing that the respiratory care professional faces the task of working with a seemingly endless number of formulas and reference values, this guide includes as many of these as possible in the most useful form. To that end, all formulas are expressed in their classical forms as well as, whenever possible, their newer variations.

Information unfolds logically and progressively in nine chapters. Chapters 1 through 4 cover the basics: medical gas therapy, physiologic monitoring, lab work, and respiratory pathophysiology. Chapter 5 offers thorough, up-to-date coverage of airways and ventilators. Special coverage of home care, neonatal and pediatric care, and respiratory pharmacology is offered in Chapters 6 through 8. The concluding chapter on medical terminology is specifically designed to meet the needs of the respiratory care professional.

Eye-catching headings and an extensive index help the reader find information quickly. Ample space for recording notes is provided at the end of each chapter. Finally, the Appendices summarize commonly-referred-to information on units of measurement and offer a unique five-language interpreter.

J.H.R.

Acknowledgments

I would like to express my gratitude to Harold, Fran, and Danielle Riggs for their support during the years of my life that were in turmoil, always reminding me that when a door closes a window opens. To Susan Warner: my sincerest gratitude and love, for without her, this text could not have been completed.

It is impossible to acknowledge all of the colleagues whose influence helped shape this book. Yet I would like to single out Harold B. Surkin, friend, adviser, and colleague. All my thanks go to the following reviewers: Elizabeth Begley, R.R.T., A.A.F., Northern Virginia Community College; Robert Delorme, M.Ed., R.R.T., R.C.P., Gwinnett Area Technical College; Philip Geronimo, R.R.T., University of Toledo Community and Technical College; Thomas Hon, R.R.T., Western Pennsylvania Hospital; Allen H. Marangoni, M.M.Sc., R.R.T., Wheeling College; Jerry Mick, R.R.T., Charleston Area Medical Center; Michael McDonald, B.S., R.R.T., Ambulatory Services of America, Little Rock; and Margaret Traband, R.R.T., University of Toledo Community and Technical College. I am very much indebted to them for their tireless reading of the many drafts of the manuscript.

A special thank you goes to Jean-François Vilain, Senior Editor, and his colleagues at F.A. Davis, Judy Ilov, Philip Ashley, Zena Sandler Gordon, and Herbert J. Powell, Jr., for their hard work in putting together *Respiratory Facts*.

Finally, to all my students who, with all their questions, can only make me a better therapist and educator, my deepest thanks.

Contents

1   **Medical Gas Therapy**

GAS LAWS

Gas physics play a major role in the field of respiratory therapy. The following is a summary of the major gas laws.

Boyle's Law

If temperature and mass remain constant, the volume of a gas will vary inversely with the pressure that is applied to that gas.

Practical Application

When finding tubing compliance.

$$P_1 V_1 = P_2 V_2$$

Solve for Boyle's law for P_2 or V_2:

$$P_2 = \frac{P_1 \cdot V_1}{V_2} \text{ and } V_2 = \frac{P_1 \cdot V_1}{P_2}$$

Charles' Law

If pressure is held constant, the volume of a gas will change directly with the temperature of that gas.

Practical Application

The difference of a volume of gas at room temperature and that same gas volume at body temperature.

To solve Charles' law for temperature and volume:

$$\frac{V_1}{T_1} = \frac{V_2}{T_2}$$

$$T_2 = \frac{T_1 \cdot V_1}{V_2} \text{ and } V_2 = \frac{V_1 \cdot T_2}{T_1}$$

Avogadro's Law

If pressure and the temperature of a gas remain constant, equal volumes of a gas will contain the same number of molecules. This number is 6.02×10^{23} molecules per gram molecular weight (gmw) of gas. The molar volume is 22.4 L at 0°C and 76 cmHg pressure.

Because of Avogadro's observation, the method of measuring the densities of a gas has been simplified.

Practical Application

The density of a given gas may be found.

$$D = \frac{\text{gmw of the gas}}{22.4 \text{ L}}$$

The answer is read as densities in g/L.

$$D \, O_2 = \frac{32}{22.4} = 1.43 \text{ g/L}$$

Gay-Lussac's Law

If volume is constant, the pressure of the gas will vary directly with absolute temperature.

Practical Application

Safety release systems for pressure. If the temperature increases, the pressure in the system will be vented to room air.

Gay-Lussac's Law is written:

$$\frac{P_1}{T_1} = \frac{P_2}{T_2}$$

To solve for pressure when volume and mass are constant:

$$P_2 = \frac{P_1 \cdot T_2}{T_1}$$

Combined Gas Law

Pressure, temperature, and volume of a gas are related if the amount of gas remains constant:

$$\frac{P_1 \cdot V_1}{T_1} = \frac{P_2 \cdot V_2}{T_2}$$

Ideal Gas Law

Apply to dilute gases at temperatures above the gases' boiling point, which demonstrates interrelationships among volume, temperature, pressure, and the amount of gas:

$$PV = {}_nRT$$

Dalton's Law

Also known as Dalton's law of partial pressure, states that the total pressure of a gas mixture is equal to the sum of the partial pressure of each gas. If you know the percentage of a certain gas in a mixture and then multiply the total pressure, you could find the partial pressure of a certain gas.

Practical Application

Used to find partial pressure of a gas; also used to calculate alveolar gas partial pressure:

$$P_x = P \cdot F_x \quad \text{or} \quad P_{tot} = P_1 + P_2 + P_3 + P_4. \ldots$$

where P_x = partial pressure of a gas
  P = pressure, usually total atmospheric barometric pressure
  F = fractional concentration of gas (x)

Poiseuille's Law

That pressure through a tube is directly proportional to the gas flow rate. This will show the degree of resistance for fluid or flow through a tube and is directly related to length, flow, and viscosity. It is inversely related to the fourth power of the radius of the tube. Poiseuille's law is written:

$$\text{Flow cm}^3/\text{sec} = \Delta P \, \frac{\pi r^4}{8 \, nl} \quad \text{or} \quad \Delta P = \frac{\dot{V}}{r^4}$$

where $\dot{V}$ = flow cm^3/sec
  ΔP = pressure gradient $(P_1 - P_2)$ from proximal to distal end of a tube
  L = length (cm)
  r = radius
  nl = viscosity
  π = 3.1416

Reynolds' Number

Clinically rarely used. Deals with laminar flow and turbulent flow of a gas through a tube. The magic number is 2000. If calculations are lower than 2000, it is said to be *laminar flow*; if greater than 2000, it is said to be *turbulent flow*. Reynolds' number is determined using the equation:

$$\frac{\text{Critical velocity (cm/sec) radius (cm) density (g/cm}^3)}{\text{Viscosity}}$$

Bernoulli Theorem

As the forward velocity of a gas increases, its lateral wall pressure decreases with a corresponding increase in forward pressure.

Practical Application

Air entrainment mask.

Henry's Law
Graham's Law
Fick's Law

All three laws deal with diffusion.

Henry's Law

The concentration of a gas dissolving in a liquid at a given temperature is proportional to the partial pressure of the gas. Simply stated, the higher the pressure the more it will dissolve at a given temperature.

$$C = K \cdot P_x$$

Graham's Law

The rate of diffusion of a gas is inversely proportional to its molecular weight. The lighter the gas, the more quickly it diffuses.

Diffusibility of gas x when compared with gas y would read:

$$\text{Diffusibility of a gas} = \frac{\text{sol coef (x)} \sqrt{\text{gmw(y)}}}{\text{sol coef (y)} \sqrt{\text{gmw(x)}}}$$

Fick's Law

The rate of diffusion of gases in a medium is proportional to the gradient of their concentration.

$$\text{Diffusibility} = C_1 - C_2$$

where C = the concentration of a gas will move from an area of higher concentration to an area of lower concentration

Law of Laplace

States the difference between the pressure on the inside of a sphere versus that on the outside is dependent on the surface tension of the air/liquid interface and the size (radius) of the bubble. The law of Laplace is written:

$$P = \frac{2_T}{R}$$

where P = pressure difference between inside/outside
T = surface tension
R = radius of sphere

OXYGEN ADMINISTRATION

Entrainment Equations

The following equations can be used to find fractional concentration of inspired oxygen (FI_{O_2}), O_2 flow, air flow, and total flow.

$$FI_{O_2} = \frac{O_2 \text{ flow} + (0.21 \times \text{air flow})}{\text{Total flow}}$$

or

$$FI_{O_2} = .21 + \frac{(.79 \times O_2 \text{ flow})}{\text{Total flow}}$$

$$O_2 \text{ flow} = \text{total flow} \times \frac{(FI_{O_2} - .21)}{.79}$$

$$\text{Air flow} = \text{total flow} - O_2 \text{ flow}$$

$$\text{Total flow} = \frac{O_2 \text{ flow} \times .79}{FI_{O_2} - .21}$$

$$\frac{\text{Air flow}}{\text{O}_2 \text{ flow}} \text{ ratio} = \frac{1.0 - \text{FI}_{\text{O}_2}}{\text{FI}_{\text{O}_2} - .21}$$

Magic Box

Another quick method to find total flow, air to oxygen ratio, and air to oxygen flow is called the *magic box* (Fig. 1–1).

Draw a box and place 100 at the top left and 21 (20 can be used with $\text{FI}_{\text{O}_2} > 30\%$) at the bottom left. Place the percentage you are looking for in the middle of the box, subtract from upper left to lower right, then from lower left to upper right. The number that is on the top is oxygen, the number on the bottom is air. You should now have a ratio. Oxygen is always 1, while air will vary with percentage. If the oxygen flow meter is set at 15 L, the air flow meter must be set at 15 L to obtain 40%; adding the two flows together, you can find the total flow, which in this case is 20 L/minute, 5 L of oxygen plus 15 L of air.

The magic box can also be done in the following manner (Fig. 1–2): by placing 100% and 21% at the top corners of the box, and the desired FI_{O_2} in the middle, simple subtraction will give you a ratio. If you know what the oxygen is set on, you can find total flow by multiplying the air ratio with the oxygen flow.

High-Flow Oxygen Systems

High-flow oxygen systems are those that meet or exceed the patient's total flow demands, also known as *peak flow*.

Normal peak flow = 4 × respiratory rate × tidal volume

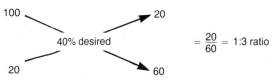

Figure 1–1. Magic Box. Subtract percentage you want from oxygen and air, and then place in a ratio.

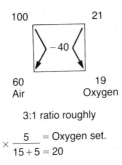

3:1 ratio roughly

$$\times \frac{5}{15+5} = 20 = \text{Oxygen set.}$$

Air is set 15 liters per minute, oxygen at 5 liters per minute
This Short Cut Works for Most FIO_2 <u>EXCEPT</u> for <u>30%</u>.

Figure 1-2. Magic box problem worked out for total flow and liter settings for an FI_{O_2} of 40%.

or

Peak flow $= (I_t + E_t/time)$ (respiratory rate) (tidal volume)

The devices that can meet or exceed patient demand (Table 1-1):

Venturi mask: Liter flow varies with percentage of O_2; most Venturi masks have FI_{O_2} from 24% to 50%.

Nebulizer with mask: a reservoir placed distal to the patient will

Table 1-1. AIR ENTRAINMENT RATIOS FOR VENTURI MASKS AND NEBULIZERS

O_2 %	Air		Oxygen
24	25	:	1
28	10	:	1
30	8	:	1
35	5	:	1
40	3	:	1
50	1.7	:	1
60	1	:	1
70	0.6	:	1
80	0.3	:	1

help prevent entrainment of ambient air when using a mask, or Tee-piece.

Tee-Piece (Briggs): Can deliver precise O_2 with high humidity, which can be cool or heated. FI_{O_2} ranges from 24% to 100%. With some types of aerosol bottles you may need more than one nebulizer set up for FI_{O_2} above 50%. Liter flow ranges from 8 to 12 L/minute or higher for these high-flow devices.

Low-Flow Oxygen Systems

Low-flow oxygen systems (Table 1-2) are devices that do not meet the patient's inspiratory demand, so room air is or can be entrained through the mouth or nose; the normal anatomical reservoir in adults is about 50 ml.

Indications

Low-flow oxygen systems are indicated for patients with tidal volumes 300 to 700 ml, respiratory rate less than 25 breaths per minute, normal breathing pattern, and arterial blood gases within normal limits on prescribed liter flow.

FI_{O_2}s on low-flow systems are not exact because they depend on the patient's depth, rate, and volume of each breath.

Approximate FI_{O_2} levels for nasal cannulas are presented in Table 1-3.

Table 1-2. LOW-FLOW DEVICES

Device	Liter Flow*	% O_2 Delivered
Nasal catheter	½-6 L/minute	23%/50%
Nasal cannula	½-6 L/minute	23%/50%
Simple mask	6-8 L/minute	40%/50%
Partial rebreather mask	6-15 L/minute	50%/80%
Non-rebreather mask	6-15 L/minute	70%/100%

*Liter flow varies according to different sources. FI_{O_2} varies with patient rate and tidal volume.

Table 1-3. APPROXIMATE FI_{O_2} LEVELS
FOR NASAL CANNULAS

Flow	FI_{O_2}
1 L/minute	0.24
2 L/minute	0.28
3 L/minute	0.32
4 L/minute	0.36
5 L/minute	0.40
6 L/minute	0.44

Flow above 6 L/minute is not recommended because drying of the mucous membrane may occur.

OXYGEN THERAPY EQUIPMENT AND MATERIALS

Gas Cylinders

Cylinders can be manufactured from non–heat-treated or heat-treated steel and aluminum, or they can be spun or stamped from steel, chrome molybdenum, or aluminum.

The Department of Transportation (DOT) governs the transportation, testing, and construction of cylinders. The National Fire Protection Agency (NFPA) sets standards for fire codes and methods of enforcing these codes. The Compressed Gas Association (CGA) is a board of representatives from hospitals, industry, and government that developed safety regulations.

Gases

The gases that are placed in these cylinders are divided into medical, laboratory, anesthetics, flammable, and nonflammable and those gases that support combustion (Table 1-4). The flammability and use of different gases are presented in Table 1-5.

Cylinder Sizes and Filling Information

These are presented in Table 1-6.

Table 1-4. TYPES OF GASES

Laboratory Gases
   Carbon dioxide (CO_2)
   Helium (He)
   Nitrogen (N_2)

Therapy Gases
   Air
   Helium-oxygen (He/O_2)
   Oxygen (O_2)
   Oxygen-carbon dioxide (O_2/CO_2)
   Oxygen-nitrogen (O_2/N_2)

Anesthetics
   Cyclopropane $(CH_2)_3$
   Ethylene (C_2H_4)
   Nitrous oxide (N_2O)

Flammable Gases
   Ethylene and cyclopropane

Nonflammable Gases
   Nitrogen, carbon dioxide, and helium

Combustion-Supporting Gases
   Oxygen
   Helium/oxygen
   Oxygen/nitrogen
   Oxygen/carbon dioxide
   Nitrous oxide

Oxygen, Air, and Nitrogen Cylinder Filling Information

   This information is presented in Table 1-7.

Tank Label Information
Contents
Instructions in case of accidental exposure
Hazards and warnings
Purity of the gas
Chemical name and letters

Table 1–5. FLAMMABILITY AND USE
OF DIFFERENT GASES

Gas	Flammability	Use
Oxygen (O_2)	Supports combustion	Therapy
Air (O_2/N_2)	Supports combustion	Therapy
Carbon dioxide (CO_2)	Nonflammable	Laboratory
Carbon dioxide–oxygen (CO_2/O_2)	Supports combustion	Therapy
Nitrogen (N_2)	Nonflammable	Laboratory
Helium (He)	Nonflammable	Laboratory
Helium–oxygen (He/O_2)	Supports combustion	Therapy
Nitrous oxide (N_2O)	Supports combustion	Anesthesia
Cyclopropane ($CH_2)_3$	Flammable	Anesthesia
Ethylene (C_2H_4)	Flammable	Anesthesia

Color Coding for E Cylinders

This is presented in Table 1–8.

Cylinder Markings
Service pressure
DOT specification
Hydrostatic test dates
Retest pass marks + or ★

Table 1–6. SIZES OF CYLINDERS

Type*	Diameter (inches)	Height (inches)	Weight (lb)
A	3	10	2½
B	3½	16	5¼
D	4¼	20	10¼
E	4½	30	15
M	7	47	66
G	8½	55	98
H&K	9	55	100

*Letters indicate cylinder size.

Table 1–7. OXYGEN, AIR, AND NITROGEN CYLINDER FILLING INFORMATION

Size Tank	Cubic Feet	Liters
D	12.6	356.0
E	22.0	622.0
M	106.0	3028.0
G	186.0	5260.0
H&K	244.0	6900.0

Inspector's mark
Serial number
Ownership mark
Manufacturer's mark
Elastic expansion number

Table 1–8. COLOR CODING FOR E CYLINDERS

Gas	United States	International
Oxygen	Green	White
Air	Yellow/silver	White/black
Carbon dioxide	Gray	Gray
Carbon dioxide – oxygen*	Gray/green	Gray/white
Helium	Brown	Brown
Helium – oxygen*	Brown/green	Brown/white
Nitrous oxide	Blue	Blue
Cyclopropane	Orange	Orange
Ethylene	Red	Violet

*Proportions of color on cylinders are roughly equivalent to the proportions of gas within the cylinder.

IT SHOULD BE NOTED THAT COLOR CODES ARE REQUIRED FOR ONLY E CYLINDERS; SOME LARGER TANKS USE THE SAME COLORS. READ THE LABEL FIRST.

Cylinder Valve Connection Safety Systems

American Standard Safety System (ASSS). Used for high-pressure systems over 200 psig. Indexed for thread type, thread size, right- or left-handed threading, external or internal threading, and nipple seat design.

Diameter Index Safety System (DISS). Used for low-pressure systems under 200 psig. Indexed for thread type, thread size, right- or left-handed threading, external or internal threading, and nipple seat design.

Pin Index Safety System (PISS). Used for E, A, and D cylinders, using a yoke connection with two prearranged pins for a specific gas.

Listing for PISS Connections for Different Gases.
Air, 1 – 5
Oxygen, 2 – 5
Carbon dioxide under 7%, 2 – 6
Helium – oxygen, 2 – 4
Ethylene, 1 – 3
Nitrous oxide, 3 – 5
Cyclopropane, 3 – 6
Carbon dioxide over 7%, 1 – 6

High-Pressure Systems

Cylinder, piping systems, and bulk oxygen systems that have higher than 200 psig of pressure in them.

Low-Pressure Systems

Devices that use pressures that have been reduced to under 200 psig.

Duration of Cylinders

To find tank factors:

$$K \ (L/psi) = \frac{\text{Volume of gas in a full tank (in cubic feet)} \times 28.3 \ L/\text{cubic foot}}{\text{Pressure of a full tank (psig)}}$$

For example, an E cylinder contains 22.0 cubic feet of gas, with a filling pressure of 2200 psig.

$$K = \frac{22.0 \times 28.3}{2200} = \frac{622.6}{2200} = .283,$$

which is the factor for E tanks

For proper units see the first equation; the units were left out of the example for the sake of simplicity.

The known factor of 28.3 L/cubic foot is the conversion of cubic feet to liters. Once (K) is found, you can find cylinder duration time.

$$\frac{(K) \times (\text{pressure read on gauge})}{\text{Liter flow the patient is on}} = \text{Time in minutes remaining}$$

To convert minutes to hours, divide by 60. For example, given an E cylinder with 2200 psig running at 2 L/minute, how long will it last?

$$\frac{.28 \times 2200}{2 \ L} = 308 \text{ minutes}$$

308 minutes divided by 60 sec = 5.13 hours

.13 hours × 60 = 7.8 minutes

This cylinder will last 5 hours and 7 minutes.

It should be noted that you do not round numbers up; if you did you would be out of oxygen.

K Factors for Cylinders

This information is presented in Table 1–9.

Table 1-9. K FACTORS FOR
CYLINDER DURATION

Gas	Cylinder Size			
	D	*E*	*G*	*H&K*
O₂,Air	0.16	0.28	2.41	3.14
O₂/CO₂	0.20	0.35	2.94	3.84
He/O₂	0.14	0.23	1.93	2.50

Liquid Oxygen Systems

A conversion chart for liquid oxygen, such as the ones shown in Tables 1-10, 1-11, and 1-12, is the only way to determine the durations of different volumes of liquid oxygen used in home oxygen care. At this time there are a number of sizes of liquid systems that are used in the home.

By obtaining a content gauge reading (from liquid system) and matching the liter flow the patient is on, you can obtain an estimate of how long the system will last in days and hours.

USAGE OF OXYGEN THERAPY

The physiological reasons for oxygen therapy using high-flow or low-flow systems are to relieve hypoxia, thereby decreasing the work of breathing and the work of the heart. By administering oxygen and reducing hypoxia, one may be able to relieve peripheral vasodilatation, pulmonary vasoconstriction, and tachycardia.

Hypoxia

Ventilation/perfusion mismatching and true shunting are the most common causes of hypoxia.

Hypoxemic Hypoxia

This is caused by inadequate arterial blood oxygen tension, as with high altitudes, sometimes called *mountain sickness,* and hypoventilation.

Table 1–10. CONVERSION CHART FOR LIQUID OXYGEN SYSTEM: 18-LITER TANK*

Contents Gauge Reading	1	2	3	4	5
Liquid Weight (lb)	5½	11¼	22½	33¾	45¼
Liquid Liters	2¼	4½	9	13½	18
Gaseous Liters	1936	3872	7745	11618	15490
Liters/Minute	**Duration Periods†**				
.5	2½ D	5¼ D	10¾ D	16 D	21½ D
1	1¼ D	2½ D	5¼ D	8 D	10¾ D
1.5	21 H	1¾ D	3½ D	5¼ D	7 D
2	16 H	1¼ D	2½ D	4 D	5¼ D

	12 H	1 D	2 D	3 D	4¼ D
2.5	12 H	1 D	2 D	3 D	4¼ D
3	10 H	21 H	1¾ D	2½ D	3½ D
3.5	9 H	18 H	1½ D	2¼ D	3 D
4	8 H	16 H	1¼ D	2 D	2½ D
4.5	7 H	14 H	28 H	1¾ D	2¼ D
5	6 H	12 H	25 H	1½ D	2 D
6	5 H	10 H	21 H	1¼ D	1¾ D
7	4½ H	9 H	18 H	27 H	1½ D
8	4 H	8 H	16 H	24 H	1¼ D

*All figures are approximate and are based on continual use.
†D = days, H = hours
(From Mid-Atlantic Health Assoc. Inc., McKeesport, PA, 1987, with permission.)

Table 1-11. CONVERSION CHART FOR LIQUID OXYGEN SYSTEM: 28-LITER TANK*

Contents Gauge Reading	1	2	3	4	5
Liquid Weight (lb)	8¾	17½	35	52¾	70¼
Liquid Liters	3½	7	14	21	28
Gaseous Liters	3012	6024	12048	18073	24097
Liters/Minute			**Duration Periods†**		
.5	4 D	8¼ D	16½ D	25 D	33¼ D
1	2 D	4 D	8¼ D	12½ D	16½ D
1.5	1¼ D	2¾ D	5½ D	8¼ D	11 D
2	25 H	2 D	4 D	6¼ D	8¼ D

	20 H	1½ D	3¼ D	5 D	6½ D
2.5	20 H	1½ D	3¼ D	5 D	6½ D
3	16½ H	1¼ D	2¾ D	4 D	5½ D
3.5	14½ H	28 H	2¼ D	3½ D	4¾ D
4	12½ H	25 H	2 D	3 D	4 D
4.5	11 H	22 H	1¾ D	2¾ D	3½ D
5	10 H	20 H	1½ D	2½ D	3¼ D
6	8¼ H	16½ H	1¼ D	2 D	2¾ D
7	7 H	14½ H	28 H	1¾ D	2¼ D
8	6¼ H	12½ H	25 H	1½ D	2 D

*All figures are approximate and are based on continual use.
†D = days, H = hours
(From Mid-Atlantic Health Assoc. Inc., McKeesport, PA, 1987, with permission.)

Table 1-12. CONVERSION CHART FOR LIQUID OXYGEN SYSTEM: 40-LITER TANK*

Contents Gauge Reading	1	2	3	4	5
Liquid Weight (lb)	12½	25	50	75	100
Liquid Liters	5	10	20	30	40
Gaseous Liters	4303	8606	17212	25818	34424
Liters/Minute		**Duration Periods†**			
.5	5¾ D	11¾ D	23¾ D	35¾ D	47¾ D
1	2¾ D	5¾ D	11¾ D	17¾ D	23¾ D
1.5	1¾ D	3¾ D	7¾ D	11¾ D	15¾ D
2	1¼ H	2¾ D	5¾ D	8¾ D	11¾ D

	1 D	2¼ D	4¾ D	7 D	9½ D
2.5	1 D	2¼ D	4¾ D	7 D	9½ D
3	23 H	1¾ D	3¾ D	5¾ D	7¾ D
3.5	20 H	1½ D	3¼ D	5 D	6¾ D
4	17 H	1¼ D	2¾ D	4½ D	5¾ D
4.5	15 H	1¼ D	2½ D	3¾ D	5¼ D
5	14 H	1 D	2¼ D	3½ D	4¾ D
6	11 H	23 H	1¾ D	2¾ D	3¾ D
7	10 H	20 H	1½ D	2½ D	3¼ D
8	8 H	17 H	1¼ D	2 D	2¾ D

*All figures are approximate and are based on continual use.
†D = days, H = hours
(From Mid-Atlantic Health Assoc. Inc., McKeesport, PA, 1987, with permission.)

23

Anemic Hypoxia

This can be caused by anemia or carbon monoxide poisoning. Carbon monoxide poisoning can sometimes be corrected by oxygen therapy, and the administration of 100% oxygen is the treatment of choice. Anemia requires an increase in hemoglobin content. Oxygen therapy alone will not help anemic hypoxia, but when used in combination with hyperbaric therapy, relief may be obtained.

Stagnant Hypoxia

This is caused by poor circulation, usually when heart failure and shock are present. By increasing cardiac output and restoring circulation, this type of hypoxia can be relieved.

Histotoxic Hypoxia

This occurs when the tissues are unable to accept oxygen from the blood. Administering high percentages of oxygen may correct this type of hypoxia, which is caused by poisons such as cyanide.

Determining the Effective Use of Oxygen

In determining the effective use of oxygen, we can use two terms to explain the effects seen or not seen in the patient.

The first term, *refractory hypoxemia,* can be used when oxygen is given to the patient and there is a negligible increase in the Pa_{O_2}. This is the result of true shunting and can be shown by increasing the FI_{O_2} by .20% and seeing less than a 10 mmHg increase in Pa_{O_2}, or if the patient is on .50% or more and Pa_{O_2} is less than 60 mmHg, the patient is said to have refractory hypoxia.

The second term, *responsive hypoxemia,* is used when oxygen is given to the patient and there is an increase in Pa_{O_2}. Responsive hypoxia is caused by ventilation/perfusion inequalities.

Oxygen Toxicity

Oxygen toxicity is caused by an increase in oxygen concentrations above 50% to 60%. Symptoms such as substernal pain, an occasional cough, burning pain on inspiration, and dyspnea have been seen in patients with oxygen toxicity and may occur anywhere from 3 to 60 hours after the administration of oxygen. The degree of toxicity is related more to the tension of oxygen than to the percentage of oxygen being given, as shown in space flights where the crew was given 100% oxygen for two to four weeks, which was tolerated for this period of time. It should be noted that due to the decrease in barometric pressure during the space flights, the tension was 250 mmHg, and not 760 mmHg.

Exudative Phase

In the *early* or *acute exudative phase* of oxygen toxicity, type I epithelial cells become swollen and then fragment. Alveolar congestion and interstitial edema develop.

Proliferative Phase

In the *late* or *chronic proliferative phase* of oxygen toxicity, type II epithelial cells proliferate up to nine times the normal number. Surfactant production is decreased along with the ability of alveolar macrophages to kill bacteria in the alveoli. During this time septal cells proliferate and collagen fibers appear in the interstitium. The increase in oxygen concentration leads to absorption atelectasis, alveolar collapse, oxygen pneumonia, and thickening of the alveolar septa.

BIBLIOGRAPHY

The works listed below are also suggested readings that will give the reader more information concerning the chapter content.

Abels, LF: Mosby's Manual of Critical Care. CV Mosby, St. Louis, 1979.

Burton, GG: Respiratory Care: A Guide to Respiratory Therapy. JB Lippincott, Philadelphia, 1984.

Eubanks, D: Comprehensive Respiratory Care: A Learning System. CV Mosby, St. Louis, 1985.

Kacmarck, RM: The Essentials of Respiratory Therapy, ed 2. Year Book Medical Publishers, Chicago, 1985.

McPherson, SP: Respiratory Therapy Equipment, ed 3. CV Mosby, St. Louis, 1985.

Spearman, CB: Egan's Fundamentals of Respiratory Therapy. CV Mosby, St. Louis, 1982.

NOTES

NOTES

2 **Physiologic Monitoring**

Physiologic monitoring in respiratory care has become an enviable tool to the practitioner in the clinical setting. The effects of therapy can be seen directly on the monitor, and therapy can be changed to meet the needs of the patient, with little time lost. There are a number of equations in this chapter that can aid the practitioner in the care of patients.

The reader will find there are a number of ways of using the equations and just as many ways of writing them. Incorporated into the chapter are as many different ways to write the same equation as possible.

NORMAL VALUES AND UNITS

The formulas for the values given in Table 2–1 may be found on the following pages.

PHYSIOLOGIC MONITORING

Nonhemodynamic

Respiratory Quotient

The respiratory quotient is the ratio of CO_2 production to O_2 consumption. Normal is 0.8 to 0.85. The metabolic rate will change with different types of diet: fats will change the respiratory quotient to 0.7, proteins to 0.8, and glucose to 1.0.

Respiratory quotient =

$$\frac{\text{Volume of carbon dioxide produced/minute}}{\text{Volume of oxygen consumed/minute}}$$

$$RQ = \frac{VCO_2}{VO_2}$$

Respiratory Exchange Ratio

The respiratory exchange ratio is the volume of carbon dioxide from the pulmonary capillaries to the lung divided by the volume of oxygen from the lung into the pulmonary capillaries. Under normal circumstances the respiratory quotient and the respiratory exchange ratio are equal.

Table 2-1. NORMAL VALUES
AND UNITS

Respiratory quotient	0.80-0.85
Respiratory exchange ratio	0.8
Alveolar air equation	110 mmHg on room air at sea level
Partial pressure of O_2 in inspired air	149.73 mmHg on room air
Physiologic dead space	0.20-0.40 ml (BTPS)
Compliance	Ideal, 0.1 L/cmH$_2$O
Ventilation-to-perfusion ratio	0.8, dimensionless
Venous-to-arterial shunt	2%-5%
Alveolar-to-arterial gradient	30-50 mmHg while breathing 100% O_2
Oxygen uptake equation	Adults, 240 ml/minute
Cardiac output	4.0-8.0 L/minute
Oxygen content of blood	$Ca_{O_2} = 20$ ml/100 ml of blood $Cv_{O_2} = 15$ ml/100 ml of blood
Cardiac index	3.2 ± 0.2 L/minute/m^2 body surface area
Stroke volume	60-90 ml/beat
Systemic vascular resistance	800-1200 dynes · sec · cm^5
Pulmonary vascular resistance	50-150 dynes · sec · cm^5
Coronary perfusion pressure	60-80 mmHg
Mean arterial pressure	82-102 mmHg
Oxygen availability	520-720 ml/minute/m^2
Oxygen consumption	250 ml/minute

$$\text{Respiratory exchange ratio} = \frac{\text{Vol\% carbon dioxide produced}}{\text{Vol\% oxygen consumed}}$$

or

$$R = \frac{\text{Vol\% CO}_2}{\text{Vol\% O}_2}$$

Alveolar Air Equation

Alveolar oxygen tension is needed to work many of the respiratory problems.

$P_{A_{O_2}}$ = pressure of alveolar oxygen
P_B = barometric pressure
FI_{O_2} = fraction of inspired oxygen
Pa_{CO_2} = pressure of arterial carbon dioxide
R = respiratory quotient, usually 0.8

Clinical Form

$$P_{A_{O_2}} = [(P_B - P_{H_2O})\ FI_{O_2}] - [(Pa_{CO_2}/R)] \quad (\text{Note } R = \underline{1.2})$$

or

$$P_{A_{O_2}} = [(P_B - P_{H_2O})FI_{O_2}] - \left[\frac{Pa_{CO_2}}{R}\right] \quad (\text{Note } R = \underline{0.8})$$

Classical Form

$$P_{A_{O_2}} = [(P_B - P_{H_2O})(FI_{O_2})] - (Pa_{CO_2})[(FI_{O_2} + 1 - FI_{O_2}/R)] \quad (\text{Note } R = \underline{0.8})$$

Short Form

$$P_{A_{O_2}} = [(P_B - P_{H_2O})FI_{O_2}] - [(Pa_{CO_2} \times 1.25)]$$

or

$$P_{A_{O_2}} = (PI_{O_2}) - (Pa_{CO_2} \times 1.25)$$

Partial Pressure of Inspired Oxygen

Partial pressure of a dry gas sample:

P_B = barometric pressure
P_{H_2O} = water vapor pressure
FI_{O_2} = fraction of inspired oxygen

$$PI_{O_2} = (P_B - P_{H_2O})FI_{O_2}$$

Physiologic Dead Space (Bohr Equation)

The Bohr equation shows the volume of inspired gas not directly involved in gas exchange, sometimes called *wasted ventilation.* There are three different types: anatomic dead space, alveolar dead space, and dead space effect.

V_D = volume of dead space

Vt = tidal volume

Pa_{CO_2} = partial pressure of arterial carbon dioxide

$P_{E_{CO_2}}$ = partial pressure of mean expired carbon dioxide

To find percentage:

$$V_D/Vt = Pa_{CO_2} - P_{E_{CO_2}}/Pa_{CO_2}$$

or

$$V_D/Vt = \frac{Pa_{CO_2} - P_{E_{CO_2}}}{Pa_{CO_2}}$$

To find per breath:

$$V_D = Pa_{CO_2} - P_{E_{CO_2}}/Pa_{CO_2}(Vt)$$

or

$$V_D = \frac{Pa_{CO_2} - P_{E_{CO_2}}}{Pa_{CO_2}} \times Vt$$

By measuring tidal volumes and finding dead space you can work a number of problems:

$$V_A = Vt - V_D$$
$$Vt = V_A + V_D$$
$$V_D = Vt - V_A$$

Compliance

Compliance explains the elastic behavior of a structure by comparing the change in volume in a system with the pressure necessary to maintain that change. There are many types of compliances that can be measured: static, dynamic, chest wall (thoracic), lung (proximal to intrapleural), total (airway to body surface), and machine or tubing compliance.

C_{st} = static compliance

C_{dyn} = dynamic compliance

C_L = compliance of the lung
C_w = compliance of the chest wall
C_t = compliance of the total lung
ΔP = change in pressure
ΔV = change in volume
ΔP_{plat} = change in plateau pressure
ΔP_{aw} = change in proximal airway pressure
ΔP_{pl} = change in intrapleural pressure
ΔP_{BS} = changes in pressure at body surface area
P_{pip} = peak inspiratory pressure
PEEP = positive end-expiratory pressure
ΔV_L = change in lung volume
ΔV_w = change in volume of the chest wall

The basic problem is written:

$$C = \frac{\Delta V}{\Delta P}$$

The two following equations are used for patients on mechanical ventilators. Static (no air movement) pressure can be obtained by using inspiratory hold or by occluding the exhalation valve for a few seconds just before exhalation. The equation for static compliance is:

$$C_{st} = \frac{\Delta V}{\Delta P_{plat} - PEEP}$$

The equation for dynamic compliance is:

$$C_{dyn} = \frac{\Delta V}{\Delta P_{pip} - PEEP}$$

The following equations are used for lung compliance. The basic problem is:

$$\frac{1}{C_t} = \frac{1}{C_L} + \frac{1}{C_w}$$

Compliance of the lung:

$$C_L = \frac{\Delta V}{\Delta P_{aw} - P_{pl}}$$

Compliance of the chest wall:

$$C_w = \frac{\Delta V_w}{\Delta P_{pl} - P_{BS}}$$

Total compliance:

$$C_t = \frac{\Delta V_L}{\Delta P_{aw} - P_{BS}}$$

Tubing compliance is the system compressibility, which reflects the amount of gas lost or compressed in ventilator tubing. For every centimeter of water pressure generated by the ventilator, an amount of gas will not reach the patient; it will, however, cause the ventilator tubing to expand. The ventilator tubing compliance must then be found in order to add the lost volume back to the ventilator so that it can be delivered to the patient.

1. Set the tidal volume to 200 ml.
2. Set high-pressure limit to maximum.
3. Occlude the patient connector.
4. Record the peak pressure.
5. Tubing compliance will equal the volume setting divided by the pressure:

$$C_{tubing} = \frac{\text{Tidal volume set}}{\text{Peak pressure}}$$

6. Multiply C_{tubing} by peak pressure (average).
7. Add this amount to the tidal volume.
8. You now have an adjusted tidal volume for tubing compliance.

Ventilation-to-Perfusion Ratio

$\dot{V}_A/\dot{Q}c$, or $\dot{V}/\dot{Q}$ ratio, determines the adequacy of ventilation to pulmonary blood flow.

$\dot{V}_A$ = alveolar ventilation
$\dot{Q}c$ = pulmonary blood flow
R = respiratory exchange ratio
P_B = barometric pressure
$P_{A_{H_2O}}$ = partial pressure of alveolar water
Ca_{O_2} = content of arterial oxygen in the blood
$C\bar{v}_{O_2}$ = mixed venous oxygen content
$P_{A_{CO_2}}$ = partial pressure of alveolar carbon dioxide
Basic equation:

$$\dot{V}_A/\dot{Q}c = \frac{R\,(P_B - P_{A_{H_2O}})(Ca_{O_2} - C\bar{v}_{O_2})}{P_{A_{CO_2}} \times 100}$$

During normal ventilation and perfusion the ratio is 0.8.

Venous-to-Arterial Shunt

$\dot{Q}s/\dot{Q}t$ shows the relationship of blood shunted to total cardiac output.

$\dot{Q}s$ = volume shunt
$\dot{Q}t$ = total cardiac output
Cc_{O_2} = oxygen content of end pulmonary capillary blood
Ca_{O_2} = oxygen content of arterial blood
$C\bar{v}_{O_2}$ = oxygen content of mixed venous blood
$P_{A_{O_2}}$ = pressure of alveolar oxygen
Pa_{O_2} = pressure of arterial oxygen
$C(a - \bar{v})$ = arterial to venous content difference

Clinical Form

$$\dot{Q}s/\dot{Q}t = \frac{(P_{A_{O_2}} - Pa_{O_2})\,.003}{C(a - \bar{v})_{O_2} + (P_{A_{O_2}} - Pa_{O_2})\,.003}$$

Classical Form

$$\dot{Q}s/\dot{Q}t = \frac{Cc'_{O_2} - Ca_{O_2}}{Cc'_{O_2} = C\bar{v}_{O_2}}$$

Short Form (Estimate)

$$\dot{Q}s/\dot{Q}t = \frac{(P_{A_{O_2}} - Pa_{O_2}) \, .003}{(P_{A_{O_2}} - Pa_{O_2}) \, .003 + 3.5}$$

or

$$\dot{Q}s/\dot{Q}t = \frac{P_{(A - a)_{O_2}}}{20}$$

Alveolar-to-Arterial Oxygen Gradient

This is used to estimate the degree of intrapulmonary shunting.

$P_{(A - a)_{O_2}}$ = alveolar-to-arterial oxygen gradient (difference)
P_B = barometric pressure
P_{H_2O} = water vapor pressure
FI_{O_2} = fraction of inspired oxygen
Pa_{O_2} = pressure of arterial oxygen
Pc_{CO_2} = pressure of arterial carbon dioxide
PI_{O_2} = pressure of inspired oxygen

Equation:

$$P_{(A - a)_{O_2}} = \left[[(Pb - P_{H_2O}) \, FI_{O_2}] - \left(\frac{Pa_{CO_2}}{.8} \right) \right] - Pa_{O_2}$$

or

$$P_{(A - a)_{O_2}} = \left[PI_{O_2} - \left(\frac{Pa_{CO_2}}{.8} \right) \right] - Pa_{O_2}$$

Oxygen Uptake and Oxygen Consumption

These equations are basically equal.

CO = cardiac output
$Ca - \overline{V}_{O_2}$ = content of arterial – content of mixed venous oxygen
V_E = exhaled minute volume (ml/minute STPD)
FI_{O_2} = fraction of inspired oxygen
$F\overline{E}_{O_2}$ = fraction of oxygen in mixed exhaled gas

$F_{\bar{E}CO_2}$ = fraction of carbon dioxide in mixed exhaled gas
For $FI_{O_2} < 1.0$, the basic equation:

$$V_{O_2} = V_E[FI_{O_2}\left[\frac{1 - F_{\bar{E}CO_2} - F_{\bar{E}O_2}}{1 - FI_{O_2}}\right]] - F_{\bar{E}O_2}$$

or

For $FI_{O_2} > 1.0$, the basic equation:

$$\dot{V}_{O_2} = V_E(FI_{O_2} - F_{\bar{E}O_2})$$

or

$$\dot{V}_{O_2} = CO \times Ca - \overline{V}_{O_2}$$

Cardiac Output (Fick Principle)

Cardiac output assumes a steady state of circulation and ventilation. Increases in cardiac output can result from either an increase in heart rate or stroke volume, or both.

$\dot{Q}$ or CO = cardiac output
$\quad$ SV = stroke volume
$\quad$ HR = heart rate
$\quad$ V_{O_2} = volume in ml/minute STPD of oxygen
$\quad$ Ca_{O_2} = arterial oxygen content in ml/100 ml
$\quad$ $C\bar{v}_{O_2}$ = mixed venous oxygen content ml/100 ml
Equation:

$$CO = SV \times HR$$

or

$$\dot{Q} = \frac{\dot{V}_{O_2}}{(Ca_{O_2} - C\bar{v}_{O_2})}$$

Oxygen Content of Blood

Oxygen content is the total volume percent of oxygen carried in the blood, including that dissolved in plasma and that bound to hemoglobin. There are three types that can be figured: content arterial oxygen, content of mixed venous, and end-pulmonary capillary content.

Ca_{O_2} = arterial oxygen content

$C\bar{v}_{O_2}$ = mixed venous oxygen content

Cc'_{O_2} = end-pulmonary capillary oxygen content

Hb = hemoglobin

$P\bar{v}_{O_2}$ = partial pressure oxygen of oxygen in mixed venous blood

Pa_{O_2} = partial pressure of arterial oxygen

Pc_{O_2} = partial pressure of end-pulmonary capillary blood, sometimes assumed to equal $P_{A_{O_2}}$

Equations:

$$Ca_{O_2} = (Hb \times 1.39 \times O_2 \text{ sat}) + (0.0031 \times Pa_{O_2})$$

$$C\bar{v}_{O_2} = (Hb \times 1.39 \times O_2 \text{ sat}) + (0.0031 \times P\bar{v}_{O_2})$$

$$Cc'_{O_2} = (Hb \times 1.39 \times O_2 \text{ sat}) + (0.0031 \times Pc_{O_2})$$

Vol% O_2 content $= (Hb \times 1.39 \times O_2 \text{ sat})$

Henderson-Hasselbach Equation

The Henderson-Hasselbach equation is a simplified form of acid–base relationship in terms of the bicarbonate ion to carbonic acid ratio.

Chemical equation:

$$H_2CO_2 - H^+ + HCO_3^-$$

Basic equation:

$$-\log[H^+] = -\log Ka -\log\left(\frac{0.03\ P_{CO_2}}{HCO_3^-}\right)$$

Simple form:

$$pH = 6.1 + \log\frac{HCO_3^-}{\text{dissolved } CO_2} = 6.1 + \log\frac{\text{total } CO_2 - 0.03}{0.03\ (P_{CO_2})}$$

or

$$pH = 6.1 + \log \frac{HCO_3^-}{H_2CO_3} = 6.1 + \log \frac{HCO_3^-}{Pa_{CO_2}(0.03)}$$

Hemodynamic

Cardiac Output

Cardiac output can be determined by the thermal dilution method using the Swan-Ganz catheter. Knowing the volume of a solution injected into the Swan-Ganz catheter placed in the right atrium and knowing the temperatures of blood and the solution, you can calculate cardiac output by charting the change in temperature against time.

$\dot{Q}$ or CO = cardiac output

V = volume of a solution injected through the Swan-Ganz catheter

Tb = temperature of blood

Ts = temperature of the solution injected

Tmb = mean change in temperature of blood

t = time from appearance to disappearance of temperature change at sampling site

Equation:

$$\dot{Q} \text{ or } CO = \frac{V \cdot (Tb - Ts)}{Tmb \cdot t}$$

Cardiac Index

The cardiac output is sometimes expressed in terms of body size and is then called *cardiac index*. The cardiac index becomes important when comparing cardiac outputs of different-size people.

CI = cardiac index

CO = cardiac output

BSA = body surface area (m²)

Equation:

$$CI = \frac{CO}{BSA}$$

Stroke Volume

The stroke volume is the volume of blood that the left ventricle injects with each contraction.

SV = stroke volume
CO = cardiac output (L/minute)
HR = heart rate (beats/minute)
Equation:

$$SV = \frac{CO \times 1000}{HR}$$

Vascular Resistance

The opposition to blood flow in a vessel cannot be measured directly but can be calculated using measurements of blood flow and pressure.

R = resistance
ΔP = change in pressure
$\dot{Q}$ = cardiac output

$$R = \frac{\Delta P}{\dot{Q}}$$

Systemic Vascular Resistance

SVR = systemic vascular resistance
MAP = mean arterial pressure
CVP = central venous pressure
CO = cardiac output
Equation:

$$SVR = \frac{MAP - CVP}{CO} \times 80$$

Pulmonary Vascular Resistance

PVR = pulmonary vascular resistance

MPAP = mean pulmonary artery pressure
PAWP = pulmonary artery wedge pressure
   CO = cardiac output
Equation:

$$PVR = \frac{MPAP - PAWP}{CO} \times 80$$

Coronary Perfusion Pressure

Coronary circulation is almost a linear function of perfusion at the coronary ostium when mean aortic diastolic pressure is between 40 and 80 mmHg. Coronary arteries will collapse at pressures below 40 mmHg.
   CPP = coronary perfusion pressure
   ADP = arterial diastolic pressure
LVEDP = left ventricular end-diastolic pressure
Equation:

$$CPP = ADP - LVEDP$$

Mean Arterial Pressure

Mean arterial pressure is the average blood pressure.
MAP = mean arterial pressure
   DP = diastolic pressure
   SP = systolic pressure
Equation:

$$MAP = \frac{(2 \times DP) + (SP)}{3}$$

Oxygen Availability (Delivery)

Oxygen availability refers to the oxygen available for tissue consumption.
O_2 AV = oxygen available
   Ca_{O_2} = oxygen content of arterial blood
   CO = cardiac output

Equation:

$$O_2 \ AV = Ca_{O_2} \times CO \times 10$$

Oxygen Consumption

V_{O_2} = minimum volume of oxygen consumed ml/minute/m^2
Ca_{O_2} = content of oxygen in arterial blood
$C\bar{v}_{O_2}$ = mixed venous oxygen content
CI = cardiac index
Equation:

$$V_{O_2} = (Ca_{O_2} - C\bar{v}_{O_2}) \times CI \times 10$$

Oxygen Extraction Ratio

The oxygen extraction ratio is the amount of oxygen used compared to the amount of oxygen available. It is sometimes used as an indicator of the metabolic rate of the body.
O_2ER = oxygen extraction ratio
Ca_{O_2} = content of arterial oxygen
$C\bar{v}_{O_2}$ = mixed venous oxygen content
Equation:

$$O_2ER = \frac{(Ca_{O_2} - C\bar{v}_{O_2})}{Ca_{O_2}} \times 100$$

WHERE TO FIND INFORMATION FOR THE HEMODYNAMIC AND NONHEMODYNAMIC EQUATIONS

Table 2–2 provides this information.

CORRELATION OF PULMONARY ARTERY PRESSURE, PULMONARY CAPILLARY WEDGE (PCW) PRESSURE, AND CARDIAC INDEX (CI)

This information is presented in Table 2–3.

Table 2-2. WHERE TO GET
THE INFORMATION

$_A$-a gradient	The alveolar air equation and arterial blood gas samples
$a\text{-}\bar{v}D_{O_2}$	Mixed venous sample from Swan-Ganz and arterial blood gas sample
Ca_{O_2}	Content equation, arterial blood gas sample, and hemoglobin sample
C_{dyn} C_{st} C_{pul} C_t	Measured tidal volume by spirometer, pressure reading from manometer, if measuring lung compliance pressure reading from swallowed transducer adjusted to midesophageal position, pressure measured at the patient's mouth
CO	Swan-Ganz (Fick), O_2 consumption, Pa_{O_2} sat, mixed venous O_2 sat, $a\text{-}\bar{v}D_{O_2}$, and by thermodilution
$C\bar{v}_{O_2}$	CVP sample, or using $P\bar{v}_{O_2}$ reading from CVP, then doing calculations to find Cv_{O_2}
CVP	CVP catheter
FI_{O_2}	Analyzer
Pa_{CO_2}	Arterial blood gas sample
$P_{A_{O_2}}$	Alveolar air equation, also barometer pressure, FI_{O_2}, and arterial blood gas
P_{ECO_2}	Exhaled gas collection in a large Douglas bag
PI_{O_2}	P_B, P_{H_2O} (usually 47), and FI_{O_2}
$P\bar{v}_{O_2}$	Pulmonary artery (Swan-Ganz)
$\dot{Q}c'$	Pulmonary blood flow via Swan-Ganz
$\dot{Q}s$	Blood gas sample, alveolar air equation for short form, or mixed sample taken from Swan-Ganz
$\dot{Q}t$	Fick's equation, or thermodilution
$P\bar{v}_{O_2}$	Sample taken from Swan-Ganz
Pa_{O_2}	Arterial blood gas
P_{CO_2}	Blood gas sample if for Pa_{CO_2}; if for P_{ECO_2} gas is collected in a Douglas bag
V_D	Arterial blood gas sample, collection of expired CO_2 collected in a Douglas bag
Vt	Spirometer
V_E	Spirometer and a watch

TYPES OF PULMONARY EDEMA

These are presented in Table 2-4.

Table 2–3. CORRELATION OF PULMONARY ARTERY PRESSURE, PULMONARY CAPILLARY WEDGE (PCW) PRESSURE, AND CARDIAC INDEX (CI)

Pulmonary Artery Pressure	PCW Pressure	CI	Probable Etiology
N or ↓	↓	↓	Hypovolemia
N or ↓↑	↑	↓	Left ventricular failure (with large V waves in PCW pressure, consider acute MR or VSD)
N or ↑	N or ↑	↓	Cardiac tamponade (CVP = PAP = PCW pressure). Right ventricular infarct (CVP inappropriately ↑ for PCW pressure)
↓↑	N or ↓	↓	Pulmonary embolus
↑	N	N	COPD
N	N	↑	Hyperdynamic state (*e.g.,* thyrotoxicosis)
N or ↑	N or ↓	↓	Gram-negative sepsis

Note: N = normal, ↑ = elevated, ↓ = low, VSD = ventricular septal defect, PAP = pulmonary artery pressure, COPD = chronic obstructive pulmonary disease.

This is a highly simplified table intended to assist thought about etiologic processes in hemodynamic monitoring.

(From McIntyre, JD: Textbook of Advanced Cardiac Life Support. American Heart Association, Dallas, 1983, with permission.)

Table 2-4. TYPES OF PULMONARY EDEMA

Pulmonary Edema

Cardiogenic
PCW pressure >21 mmHg

Noncardiogenic
PCW pressure <12 mmHg

Hypo-osmotic
COP – PCW pressure
<4.0 mmHg

Excessive capillary permeability
COP – PCW pressure
>4.0 mmHg

Cardiogenic pulmonary edema can occur with a PCW pressure <21 mmHg if the COP <25 mmHg.

COP = capillary osmotic pressure.
(From McIntyre, JD: Textbook of Advanced Cardiac Life Support. American Heart Association, Dallas, 1983, with permission.)

47

ETIOLOGIES OF PULMONARY EDEMA

This information is presented in Table 2–5.

PULMONARY FUNCTION STUDIES

Lung Volume

Tidal Volume

Tidal volume (Vt) equals the amount of gas that is inhaled or exhaled during a normal breath. Normal Vt is 500 ml, or 3 ml per pound of ideal body weight.*

Inspiratory Reserve Volume

Inspiratory reserve volume (IRV) equals the maximum amount of gas that can be inspired above normal inspiration (above Vt). Normal IRV is 3,100 ml, or 3.1 L.*

Residual Volume

Residual volume (RV) equals the volume of gas remaining in the lung after a maximal exhalation. Normal RV is 1200 ml, or 1.2 L.*

Expiratory Reserve Volume

Expiratory reserve volume (ERV) equals the volume of gas that can be exhaled after a normal (Vt) exhalation. Normal ERV is 1200 ml, or 1.2 L.*

Lung Capacities

Capacities combine two or more lung volumes together to make one capacity.

---

*Normal volumes and capacities are based on statistical data from a group of individuals of the same height, age, and sex. The numbers are for a 6-foot tall, 25-year-old male.

Table 2-5. ETIOLOGIES OF PULMONARY EDEMA

Cardiogenic	Hypo-osmotic	↑ CAP Permeability
Left ventricular failure	(Effect 1° due to ↓ albumin)	Aspiration
Pump failure	Failure to make albumin	HCl, H_2O (fresh and salt)
Mitral regurgitation	Starvation	Noxious gases (SO_2, N_2O, NH_3, Cl_2)
Ventricular septal	Liver disease	
defect	Losses of albumin	Thermal injuries
Fluid overload	Renal	Oxygen toxicity
Mitral stenosis	Gastrointestinal	Pulmonary fat emboli
Severe hypertension	Acute pancreatitis	Shock lung syndrome
Neurogenic	Peritonitis	Gram-negative sepsis
High altitude	Ascites	

(From McIntyre, JD: Textbook of Advanced Cardiac Life Support. American Heart Association, Dallas, 1983, with permission.)

Total Lung Capacity

Total lung capacity (TLC) equals the total amount of all lung volumes (RV + Vt + ERV + IRV). Normal TLC is 6,000 ml, or 6.0 L.*

Vital Capacity

Vital capacity (VC) equals the amount of gas that can be exhaled after a maximal inspiration, or ERV + Vt + IRV. Normal VC is 4,800 ml, or 4.8 L.*

Inspiratory Capacity

Inspiratory capacity (IC) equals the total amount of gas that can be inspired after a normal exhalation (IRV + Vt). Normal IC is 3,600 ml, or 3.6 L.*

Functional Residual Capacity

Functional residual capacity (FRC) equals the amount of gas remaining in the lungs after a normal exhalation (RV + ERV). Normal is 2,400 ml, or 2.4 L.*

Predicted Lung Capacities and Volumes

By finding normal VC values for your patient, other predicted values may be obtained. Predicted VC may be found by using the following formulas:

For males:

$$VC = 27.63 - (0.112 \times age) \times (height\ in\ cm)$$

For females:

$$VC = 21.78 - (0.101 \times age) \times (height\ in\ cm)$$

ERV is approximately 25% of VC
IRV is approximately 75% of VC

IC is approximately 75% of VC

For males

$$FVC = 0.148 \times height - 0.025 \times age - 4.241$$

For females

$$FVC = 0.115 \times height - 0.024 \times age - 2.852$$

For males

$$FEV_1 = 0.092 \times height - 0.032 \times age - 1.260$$

For females

$$FEV_1 = 0.089 \times height - 0.025 \times age - 1.932$$

For males

$$FEF_{25\%-75\%} = 0.047 \times height - 0.045 \times age + 2.513$$

For females

$$FEF_{25\%-75\%} = 0.060 \times height - 0.030 \times age + 0.551$$

For males

$$TLC = 0.078 \text{ (height in cm)} - 7.30$$

For females

$$TLC = 0.079 \text{ (height in cm)} - 0.008 \times age - 7.49$$
$$VC = \text{about 80\% of TLC}$$
$$IC = \text{about 60\% of TLC}$$
$$FRC = \text{about 40\% of TLC}$$
$$RV = \text{about 20\% of TLC}$$
$$ERV = \text{about 20\% of TLC}$$
$$Vt = \text{about 8\%-10\% of TLC}$$

Pulmonary Mechanics

Forced vital capacity (FVC) is the volume of gas forced and rapidly exhaled after maximal expiratory effort.

Forced vital capacity timed (FVC_t) is the volume expired during a timed interval during the FVC maneuver.

Forced expiratory flow 200–1200 (FEF 200–1200) or maximal expiratory flow rate 200–1200 (MEFR 200–1200) is the average flow of gas after the first 200 ml of gas is exhaled during the FVC maneuver.

Forced expiratory flow 25%–75% ($FEF_{25\%-75\%}$) or mean forced expiratory flow rate 25–75 ($MMER_{25-75}$) is the average flow rate between the first 25% and 75% of the exhale volume slope.

Maximum voluntary ventilation (MVV) is the maximum volume of gas rapidly and deeply ventilated in a minute. This minute is figured by 15 sec × 4 or 30 sec × 2.

Pulmonary Function Tests

Flow volume loops are graphic analyses of flow generated during a forced expiratory maneuver, followed by a forced inspiratory maneuver. Flow is recorded in L/second.

Volume of isoflow is determined by superimposing over normal flow volume curves recorded by breathing a mixture of 80% helium and 20% oxygen. The volume of isoflow is recorded as a percent of FVC.

Single-breath nitrogen test for closing volumes is the lung volume at which airway closure begins and is expressed as percent of VC.

Nitrogen washout test (7-minute) is the manner in which oxygen is distributed in the lungs and is recorded as percent of nitrogen remaining in the lung after 7 minutes.

Carbon monoxide diffusion test measures all the factors that affect the diffusion of gas across the alveolar capillary membrane.

Equipment for Pulmonary Function Tests

Water-seal spirometers consist of a large bell suspended in a container of water with the open end of this bell below the surface of the water. Breathing into and out of the system moves the bell a proportional distance.

Dry-rolling spirometers consist of a piston in a cylinder that is supported by a rod resting on frictionless bearings. The piston is coupled to the cylinder wall by a plastic seal that rolls itself, rather than sliding.

Bellow-type spirometers consist of bellows that fold or unfold in response to breathing movements.

Wright respirometers (*spirometers*) consist of vanes connected to a number of gears, so that when gas moves through the device it registers a volume.

A *pneumotach* is a direct flow-sensing device with advanced electronics to integrate flow to volume.

The *X – Y recorder* is a recorder capable of accepting flow and volume inputs and graph either against time base or plotting flow against volume.

Interpretation of Pulmonary Function Tests

Decreased flows may indicate an obstructive lung disease, such as emphysema, bronchitis, asthma, bronchiectasis, or cystic fibrosis. Decreased lung volumes may indicate a restrictive disease state, such as inflammatory, cardiac, neurologic, neuromuscular, or pleural, thoracic deformities, or fibrotic lung diseases. When volume and flows are both decreased, the patient is said to have both obstructive and restrictive lung disease.

Setting Normal Limits and Grades of Impairment

These are provided in Tables 2 – 6 through 2 – 9.

ELECTROCARDIOGRAM (ECG, EKG)

ECG is a graphic record of the electrical activity of the heart, reflecting the depolarization and repolarization of the atria and ventricles (Figs. 2 – 1 and 2 – 2). The ECG cannot tell you about mechanical function, but it can give you rhythm disturbances and conduction problems of the heart.

Table 2-6. COEFFICIENTS OF VARIATION FOR VARIOUS PULMONARY FUNCTIONS

Function	c.v. Range (%)	Mean c.v. (%)	Number of Sources	Normal Limit % 100% – 1.64 c.v.
FVC	12.1 – 14.5	12.9	3	≥ 80
FEV$_1$	13.0 – 13.6	13.4	3	≥ 80
FEF$_{25\%-75\%}$	23.2 – 26.0	24.6	2	≥ 60
FEV$_1$/FVC	5.5 – 9.2	7.8	4	≥ 90
FEF$_{max}$	20.7 – 23.3	22.0	2	≥ 65
RV	18.6 – 25.8	24.8	5	≥ 60 < 140
FRC	15.0 – 24.0	18.6	5	≥ 70 < 130
TLC	10.0 – 13.7	11.2	5	≥ 80 < 120
D$_L$CO	12.3 – 20.0	15.1	3	≥ 75

c.v. = Coefficients of variation: range, mean.
(From Miller, WF: Laboratory Evaluation of Pulmonary Function. JB Lippincott, St. Louis, 1987, p 85, with permission.)

Table 2-7. GRADES OF VENTILATORY FUNCTION IMPAIRMENT

Grade of Defect	Volume Functions	Flow Functions		Clearance Index*	Diffusion Functions†
		A	B		
Normal	≥80	≥80	≥70	≥75	≥85
Mild	<80-70	<80-65	<70-60	<75-65	<85-70
Moderate	<70-55	<65-45	<60-40	<65-50	<70-50
Severe	<55-30	<45-20	<40-15	<50-35	<50-30
Extreme	<30	<20	<15	<35	<30

$A = FEF_{0-25\%,\ 50\%},\ FEV_{0.5},\ FEV_1$
$B = FEF_{25\%-75\%,\ 75\%,\ 75\%-85\%}$
*$FEV_1 \times 10/FVC$
†Based on the multiple point technique as used in our laboratory.
(From Miller, WF: Laboratory Evaluation of Pulmonary Function. JB Lippincott, St. Louis, 1987, p 85, with permission.)

Table 2–8. BREATHING NOMOGRAM*

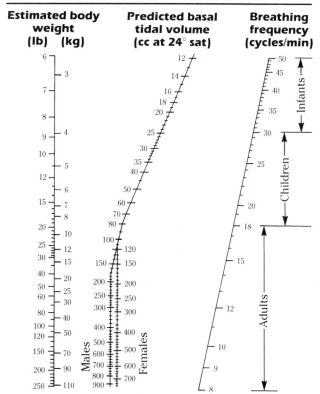

Corrections of predicted basal tidal volumes.
  For patients not in coma: add 10%
  Fever: add 5% for each °F above 99 (rectal)
         add 9% for each °C above 37 (rectal)
  Altitude: add 5% for each 2000 feet above sea level
            add 8% for each 1000 meters above sea level
  Intubation: subtract volume equal to one-half body weight in
              pounds
              subtract 1 cc/kg of body weight
  Dead space: add equipment dead space

*From Spearman, CB and Sheldon, RL: Egan's Fundamentals of Respiratory Therapy, ed 4. CV Mosby, St. Louis, 1982, p 718, with permission.

Single Cardiac Cycle

P wave: atrial depolarization

PR segment: delay in AV node

PR interval: atrial depolarization plus the delay in AV node; normally .12 to .20 second

Q wave: first negative wave after the P wave, but before the R wave; may not always be present

R wave: the first positive wave after the P wave

S wave: the negative wave after the R wave

QRS complex: may have one, two, or all three — Q,R,S; ventricular depolarization; normally .06 to .12 second

ECG Graph Paper Specifications

Time

One Small Block = .04 second

Five small blocks = .2 second

Large line or dark line = 3.0 seconds

Voltage: Size of Tracing Up and Down*

One small block = .1 mv

Ten small blocks = 1.0 mv

ECG Interpretation

Regularity (Rhythm)

Is it regular?

Is it irregular?

Are there any patterns to the irregularity?

Are there any ectopic beats?

Rate

300, 150, 100, 75, 60, 50

---

*No standardization on rhythm strips, only on 12-lead ECG.

Table 2-9. SUMMARY OF PULMONARY FUNCTION TESTS

Measurement	How Determined	Units	Disease Process	Usefulness
TLC	Body box	L and % predicted	Obstructive: ↑ → restrictive	+++
VC	Spirogram	L and % predicted	Obstructive: → ↓ restrictive	++++
ERV	Spirogram	L and % predicted	Obstructive: → ↓ restrictive	+
FRC	Derived: spirogram and body box or nitrogen washout/helium dilution	L and % predicted	Obstructive: ↑ ↓ restrictive	+++
RV	Derived: spirogram and body box or nitrogen washout/helium dilution	L and % predicted	Obstructive: ↑ ↓ restrictive	+++
TV	Spirogram	L and % predicted	↑/N obstructive: ↓ /N restrictive	++

IRV	Spirogram	L and % predicted	↓/N obstructive: ↓→/N restrictive	+
IC	Spirogram	L and % predicted	↓/N obstructive: ↓→/N restrictive	+
MVV	Spirogram	L/minute	↓ obstructive: ↓ restrictive	+++
f	Clock	Number/minute	↑ restrictive	+++
$\dot{V}E$	Derived: $f \times TV$	L/minute	↑ restrictive	+++
FEV_1	Spirogram	% predicted	↓ obstructive and restrictive	++++
FEV_3	Spirogram	% predicted	↓ obstructive and restrictive	+++
FEF_{25-75}	Spirogram	% predicted	↓ obstructive and restrictive	+++
PF	Spirogram	% predicted	↓ obstructive	++
FEV_1/FVC	Spirogram	% predicted	↓ obstructive	++++
DL_{CO_2}	Carbon monoxide uptake	% predicted	↓ emphysema and restrictive	+++
CV	Nitrogen washout	% predicted	↑ obstructive	++
Raw	Body box	% predicted	↑ obstructive	+++
Compliance	Esophageal balloon	cc/cmH$_2$O pressure	↑ obstructive: ↓ restrictive	+++

+, Least useful.

++++, Most useful.

(From Wilkins, RL: Clinical Assessment in Respiratory Care. CV Mosby, St. Louis, p 159, with permission.)

59

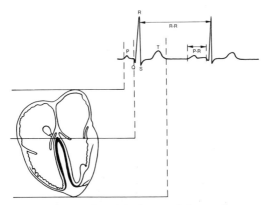

Figure 2–1. Relationship of the heart and the waveform complex. (From Brown, KR and Jacobson, S: Mastering Dysrhythmias: A Problem-Solving Guide. FA Davis, Philadelphia, 1988, p 4, with permission.)

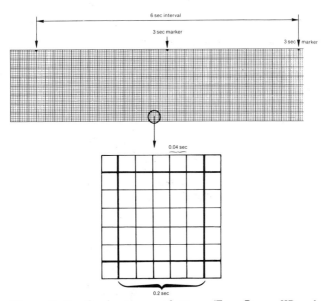

Figure 2–2. Graph paper specifications. (From Brown, KR and Jacobson, S: Mastering Dysrhythmias: A Problem-Solving Guide. FA Davis, Philadelphia, 1988, p 9, with permission.)

Count the number of QRS complexes in a 6-second strip if
  irregular.
Use a rate ruler.

P Waves

Are the P waves regular?
Is there one P wave for every QRS complex?
Is there a P wave in front of the QRS complex or behind it?
Are there more P waves than QRS complexes?

Dysrhythmias

Dysrhythmias are discussed in Tables 2–10 through
2–14 and Figures 2–3 through 2–28.

Table 2–10. COMMON
SUPRAVENTRICULAR RATES

Rhythm	Rate
Sinus tachycardia	100–150/minute
Paroxysmal supraventricular tachycardia (PSVT)	140–250/minute
Atrial flutter	250–350/minute
Atrial fibrillation	350–600/minute

(From Brown, KR and Jacobson, S: Mastering Dysrhythmias: A
Problem-Solving Guide. FA Davis, Philadelphia, 1988, with
permission.)

Table 2-11. DYSRHYTHMIA SYNOPSIS: SINUS DYSRHYTHMIAS

	P Waves	QRS Complexes	AV Relationship	Other Features
Sinus bradycardia	Normal	Normal	Normal	Rate below 60/minute
Sinus tachycardia	Normal	Normal	Normal	Rate above 100/minute
Sinus arrest/SA exit block	Missing in dropped cycles	Missing in dropped cycles	Missing in dropped cycles	Long asystolic R-R intervals during periods of arrest
	Normal in conducted cycles	Normal for conducted cycles	Normal for conducted cycles	
Sinus dysrhythmia	Normal shape	Normal shape	Normal	Benign variation of RSR
				Varies with phases of respiration
Atrial flutter	Absent, replaced by regular F waves Atrial rate of 250–350/minute	Normal Usually regular	Usually a fixed AV conduction greater than 1:1 (*e.g.,* 2:1, 3:1, 4:1)	

62

Atrial fibrillation	Absent; replaced by irregular f waves Atrial rate of 350–600/minute (not countable)	Normal Irregularly irregular; rate is under 100/minute (treated) or above 100/minute (untreated)	Random AV conduction
Multifocal atrial tachycardia	Sinus P waves plus P' waves of at least three shapes	Irregular rhythm	1 : 1
Paroxysmal supraventricular tachycardia (PSVT)	Absent P' waves are missing If present, found preceding, following, or in the QRS complex	Normal Regular R-R interval	1 : 1 if P' wave visible S2 : 1, 3 : 1 conduction, suspect digitalis toxicity
Sinus tachycardia	Normal	Normal	1 : 1
AV junctional tachycardia	Normal		

(From Brown, KR and Jacobson, S: Mastering Dysrhythmias: A Problem-Solving Guide. FA Davis, Philadelphia, 1988, with permission.)

Table 2–12. DYSRHYTHMIA SYNOPSIS: VENTRICULAR RHYTHMS

	P Waves	QRS Complexes	AV Relationship	Other Features
1. Escape idioventricular rhythm	Absent	Depends on level of escape focus High in ventricle are narrow and 40–50/minute Low in ventricle are wide and 20–40/minute	Absent	Life-sustaining in event of sinus arrest and third-degree heart block
2. Accelerated idioventricular rhythm	Absent	Wide, distorted Rate 50–100/minute	Absent or AV dissociation Occasional ventricular capture complexes	Originally thought to be benign; now considered pathologic
3. Ventricular tachycardia	Absent or sporadically present	Wide and bizarre Rate above 100/minute (commonly about 150/minute)	Absent	Resembles a string of premature ventricular contractions

4. Torsade de pointes (variation of ventricular tachycardia)	Absent	Wide and slurred QRS axis constantly changing in the same lead	Absent	Prolonged Q-T interval in normal sinus rhythm prior to or following episode of ventricular tachycardia
5. Ventricular fibrillation	Absent	No defined pattern	Absent	Chaotic tracing with complexes of varying heights and shapes
6. Asystole	Absent	Absent	Absent	Flat line

(From Brown, KR and Jacobson, S: Mastering Dysrhythmias: A Problem-Solving Guide. FA Davis, Philadelphia, 1988, with permission.)

Table 2-13. DYSRHYTHMIA SYNOPSIS: AV HEART BLOCK

	P Waves	QRS Complexes	AV Relationship	Key Features
1. First-degree	Normal All P waves are conducted	Normal No QRS complexes are dropped	P-R interval over 0.20 second Only AV block with 1:1 AV conduction	Long P-R interval Site of block within AV node
2. Second-degree A. Wenckebach type	Normal Some P waves are not conducted	Normal Some QRS complexes are dropped	Progressive increase in P-R intervals followed by dropped QRS complex Ratio typically 3:2, 4:3, etc. P-R interval of first beat in each cycle often greater than 0.20 second	Grouped beating Increasing P-R intervals The longest R-R interval is equal to less than twice the shortest one Site of blocks: intranodal
B. Mobitz type 2	Normal Some P waves are not conducted	Wide Some QRS complexes are dropped	Fixed P-R interval prior to dropped beats	Fixed P-R intervals Site of block: infranodal

			Ratio may be 3:2, 4:3 or higher degrees (4:2, 5:3, etc.) P-R interval usually normal	
3. Third-degree	Normal shape, regular intervals No P waves are conducted More P waves than QRS complexes	Escape rhythm depends on level of block Usually wide and distorted if low in ventricle Narrow if high in ventricle Regular R-R intervals Rate slower than atrial (usually below 50/minute)	Complete dissociation They are independent of one another	Site of block: infranodal AV dissociation

Note: Not all second-degree blocks with 2:1 AV conduction are type 2 blocks.
(From Brown, KR and Jacobson, S: Mastering Dysrhythmias: A Problem-Solving Guide. FA Davis, Philadelphia, 1988, with permission.)

Table 2-14. DYSRHYTHMIA SYNOPSIS: ECTOPIC COMPLEXES

	P Waves	QRS Complexes	AV Relationship	Other Features
1. Premature complexes				
A. PAC/atrial	Premature ectopic P' wave	Normal if conducted May be blocked or aberrantly conducted	1:1 AV conduction P-R interval differs from sinus complexes	Noncompensatory pause Normal T waves
B. PJC/junctional	Retrograde P' wave just before or after QRS complex Often P' wave missing	Normal	May be 1:1 or missing P-R interval often shortened	Noncompensatory pause Normal T waves
C. PVC/ventricular	Absent	Wide, bizarre	Absent	Compensatory pause Abnormal T waves (slope opposite aberrant QRS)

2. Escape complexes			
A. Atrial	P' wave	Normal	Variable	Occur in cases of sinus depression
B. Junctional	Retrograde P' wave or missing	Normal Sustained rhythm at rate of 40–60/minute	Variable	Occur when sinus node is depressed
C. Ventricular	Missing	Wide, bizarre Sustained rhythm at rate of 20–40/minute	Missing	Occur when sinus and AV junction fail as pacemaker

Notes: Premature beats occur early in the R-R interval while escape beats occur late. Premature beats compete with sinus node for pacemaker role (interrupt R-R cycles of dominant rhythm); escape beats "reluctantly" assume pacemaker role when SA node fails (end R-R cycles longer than dominant rhythm).

(From Brown, KR and Jacobson, S: Mastering Dysrhythmias: A Problem-Solving Guide. FA Davis, 1988, with permission.)

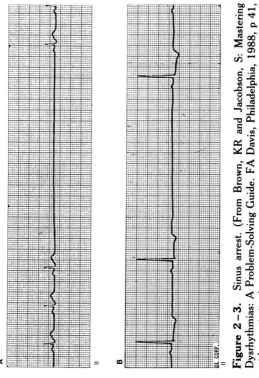

Figure 2–3. Sinus arrest. (From Brown, KR and Jacobson, S: Mastering Dysrhythmias: A Problem-Solving Guide. FA Davis, Philadelphia, 1988, p 41, with permission.)

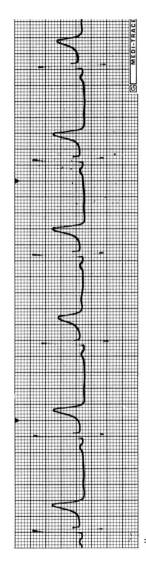

Figure 2–4. Sinus bradycardia (50/minute). (From Brown, KR and Jacobson, S: Mastering Dysrhythmias: A Problem-Solving Guide. FA Davis, Philadelphia, 1988, p 39, with permission.)

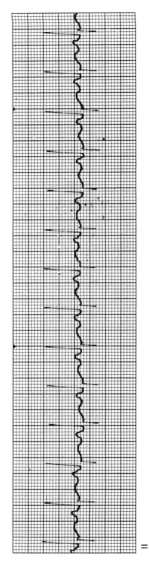

Figure 2–5. Sinus tachycardia (120/minute). (From Brown, KR and Jacobson, S: Mastering Dysrhythmias: A Problem-Solving Guide. FA Davis, Philadelphia, 1988, p 38, with permission.)

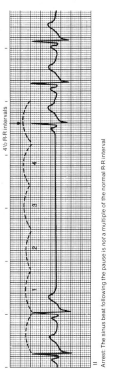

| 4½ R-R intervals |

Arrest: The sinus beat following the pause is *not* a multiple of the normal R-R interval

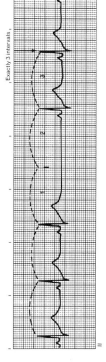

| Exactly 3 intervals |

Block: The sinus complex following the pause is an exact multiple of the normal R-R interval

t versus block.

Figure 2–6. ECG difference between sinus arrest versus block. (From Brown, KR and Jacobson, S: Mastering Dysrhythmias: A Problem-Solving Guide. FA Davis, Philadelphia, 1988, p 42, with permission.)

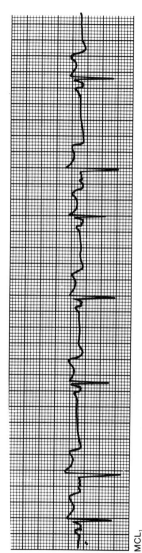

Figure 2 – 7. PACs (beats 2 and 6). (From Brown, KR and Jacobson, S: Mastering Dysrhythmias: A Problem-Solving Guide. FA Davis, Philadelphia, 1988, p 44, with permission.)

MCL₁

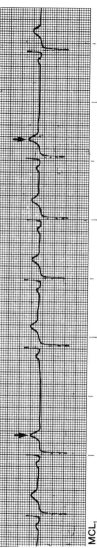

Figure 2 – 8. Nonconducted PACs. The ECG pauses are caused by the blocked P' waves (arrows), hidden in the T waves of the preceding sinus beats. (From Brown, KR and Jacobson, S: Mastering Dysrhythmias: A Problem-Solving Guide. FA Davis, Philadelphia, 1988, p 44, with permission.)

MCL₁

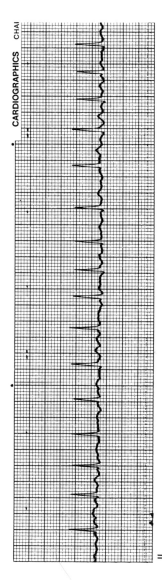

CARDIOGRAPHICS   CHAI

Figure 2–9. Atrial fibrillation with a tachycardiac (120/minute) ventricular response. (From Brown, KR and Jacobson, S: Mastering Dysrhythmias: A Problem-Solving Guide. FA Davis, Philadelphia, 1988, p 48, with permission.)

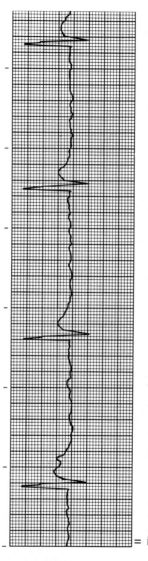

Figure 2–10. Atrial fibrillation with complete AV block. An idioventricular escape focus paces the heart at 32/minute. (From Brown, KR and Jacobson, S: Mastering Dysrhythmias: A Problem-Solving Guide. FA Davis, Philadelphia, 1988, p 49, with permission.)

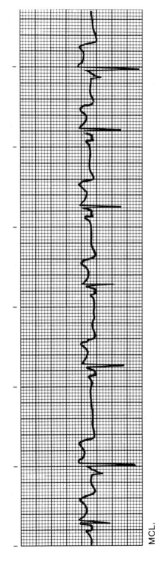

MCL₁

Figure 2–11. PJCs (beats 2 and 7). (From Brown, KR and Jacobson, S: Mastering Dysrhythmias: A Problem-Solving Guide. FA Davis, Philadelphia, 1988, p 45, with permission.)

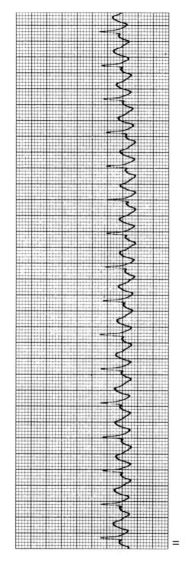

Figure 2–12. Atrial flutter with 2:1 AV conduction. (From Brown, KR and Jacobson, S: Mastering Dysrhythmias: A Problem-Solving Guide. FA Davis, Philadelphia, 1988, p 50, with permission.)

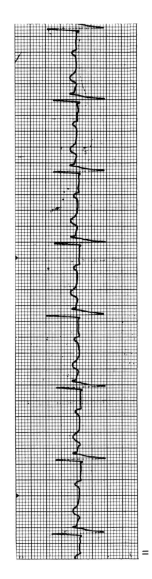

Figure 2–13. First-degree AV block (P-R interval is 0.32 sec). (From Brown, KR and Jacobson, S: Mastering Dysrhythmias: A Problem-Solving Guide. FA Davis, Philadelphia, 1988, p 88, with permission.)

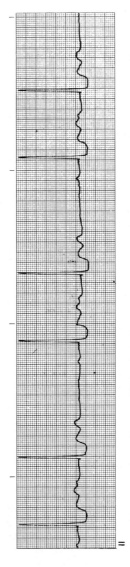

Figure 2–14. Second-degree AV block; Mobitz type 1 (Wenckebach); 3:2 AV conduction ratio. (From Brown, KR and Jacobson, S: Mastering Dysrhythmias: A Problem-Solving Guide. FA Davis, Philadelphia, 1988, p 90, with permission.)

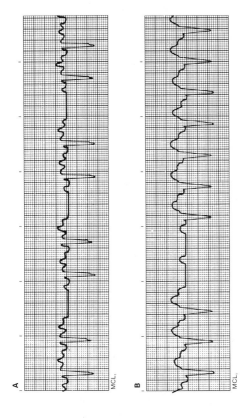

Figure 2–15. Second-degree AV blocks. *A*, Mobitz type 2, with 3:2 AV conduction. *B*, High-grade Mobitz type 2. (From Brown, KR and Jacobson, S: Mastering Dysrhythmias: A Problem-Solving Guide. FA Davis, Philadelphia, 1988, p 91, with permission.)

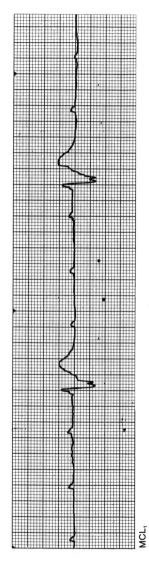

MCL₁

Figure 2-16. Third-degree (complete) AV block. (From Brown, KR and Jacobson, S: Mastering Dysrhythmias: A Problem-Solving Guide. FA Davis, Philadelphia, 1988, p 93, with permission.)

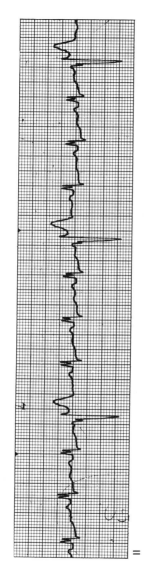

Figure 2–17. Ventricular quadrigeminy. (From Brown, KR and Jacobson, S: Mastering Dysrhythmias: A Problem-Solving Guide. FA Davis, Philadelphia, 1988, p 118, with permission.)

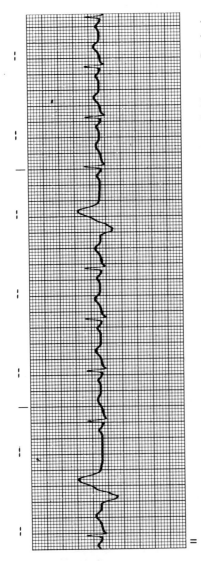

Figure 2–18. Two uniformed PVCs (beats 2 and 7). (From Brown, KR and Jacobson, S: Mastering Dysrhythmias: A Problem-Solving Guide. FA Davis, Philadelphia, 1988, p 115, with permission.)

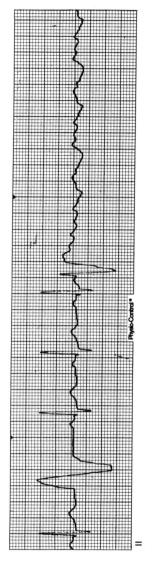

II

Figure 2–19. A PVC during the vulnerable period (T wave) causes ventricular fibrillation. (From Brown, KR and Jacobson, S: Mastering Dysrhythmias: A Problem-Solving Guide. FA Davis, Philadelphia, 1988, p 119, with permission.)

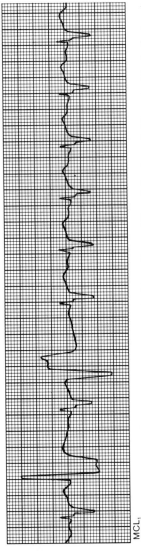

MCL₁

Figure 2–20. Multiformed PVCs (beats 2 and 4). (From Brown, KR and Jacobson, S: Mastering Dysrhythmias: A Problem-Solving Guide. FA Davis, Philadelphia, 1988, p 119, with permission.)

86

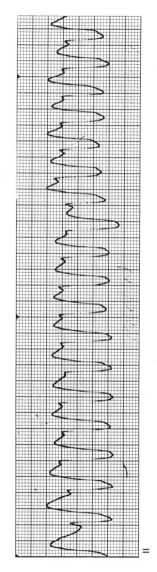

Figure 2–21. Ventricular tachycardia (160/minute). (From Brown, KR and Jacobson, S: Mastering Dysrhythmias: A Problem-Solving Guide. FA Davis, Philadelphia, 1988, p 122, with permission.)

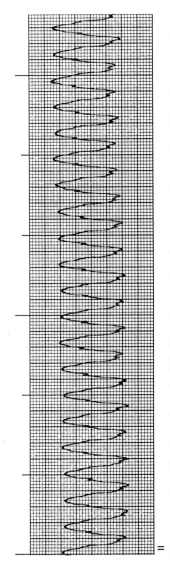

Figure 2–22. This figure shows the difficulty in distinguishing between ventricular tachycardia and supraventricular tachycardia with aberrant ventricular conduction. (From Brown, KR and Jacobson, S: Mastering Dysrhythmias: A Problem-Solving Guide. FA Davis, Philadelphia, 1988, p 122, with permission.)

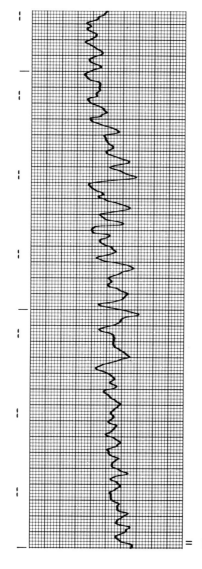

Figure 2-23. Coarse ventricular fibrillation. (From Brown, KR and Jacobson, S: Mastering Dysrhythmias: A Problem-Solving Guide. FA Davis, Philadelphia, 1988, p 127, with permission.)

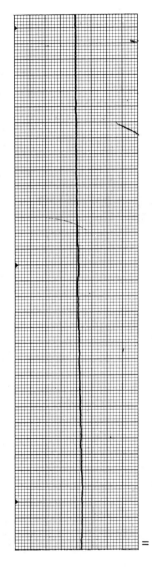

Figure 2–24. Asystole. (From Brown, KR and Jacobson, S: Mastering Dysrhythmias: A Problem-Solving Guide. FA Davis, Philadelphia, 1988, p 129, with permission.)

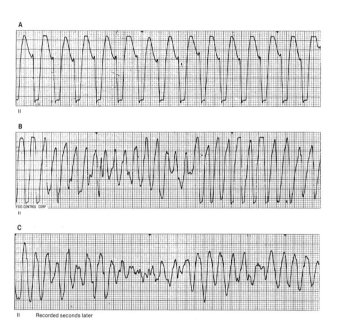

Figure 2–25. This tracing shows the fatal progression of ventricular tachycardia through periods of flutter and fibrillation. (From Brown, KR and Jacobson, S: Mastering Dysrhythmias: A Problem-Solving Guide. FA Davis, Philadelphia, 1988, p 125, with permission.)

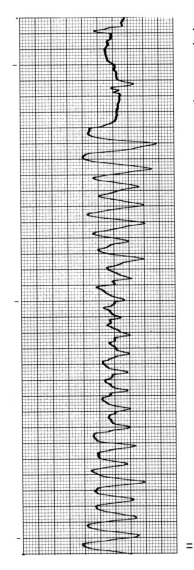

Figure 2-26. Torsade de pointes variation of ventricular tachycardia converting spontaneously to sinus rhythm. (From Brown, KR and Jacobson, S: Mastering Dysrhythmias: A Problem-Solving Guide. FA Davis, Philadelphia, 1988, p 124, with permission.)

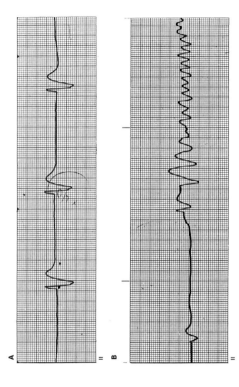

Figure 2-27. *A*, Idioventricular rhythm (30/minute). *B*, The highly unreliable nature of an idioventricular pacemaker is illustrated by this tracing. The slowly discharging focus (20/minute) degenerates into ventricular fibrillation. (From Brown, KR and Jacobson, S: Mastering Dysrhythmias: A Problem-Solving Guide. FA Davis, Philadelphia, 1988, p 126, with permission.)

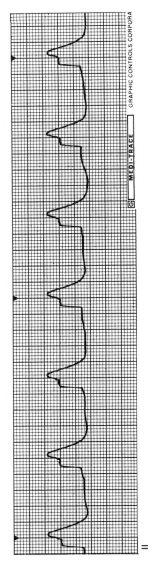

Figure 2–28. Idioventricular rhythm (accelerated at 60/minute). (From Brown, KR and Jacobson, S: Mastering Dysrhythmias: A Problem-Solving Guide. FA Davis, Philadelphia, 1988, p 126, with permission.)

94

BIBLIOGRAPHY

The works listed below are also suggested readings that will give the reader more information concerning the chapter content.

Abels, LF: Mosby's Manual of Critical Care. CV Mosby, St Louis, 1979.

Brown, KR, Jacobson, S: Mastering Dysrhythmias: A Problem-Solving Guide. FA Davis, Philadelphia, 1988.

Burton, GG: Respiratory Care: A Guide to Respiratory Therapy. JB Lippincott, Philadelphia, 1984.

Daily, EK: Techniques in Bedside Hemodynamic Monitoring, ed 3. CV Mosby, St. Louis, 1985.

Kacmarck, RM: The Essentials of Respiratory Therapy, ed 2, Year Book Medical Publishers, Chicago, 1985.

McIntyre, JD: Textbook of Advanced Cardiac Life Support. American Heart Association, Dallas, 1983.

Meter, MV, Lavine PG: Reading EKG's Correctly, Nursing Skillbook. Intermed Communications, Horsham, PA, 1975.

Miller, WF: Laboratory Evaluation of Pulmonary Function. JB Lippincott, St. Louis, 1987.

Spearman, CB: Egan's Fundamentals of Respiratory Therapy. CV Mosby, St. Louis, 1982.

NOTES

3 Lab Work

Arterial Blood Gases
    Technique
    Normal Ranges
    Interpretation
Normal Lab Values for Electrolytes,
   Hematology, Urine, and Cerebrospinal Fluid
Increases, Decreases, Causes, and Symptoms
   of Altered Lab Work
    Electrolytes
        Calcium (Ca^{++})
            Hypercalcemia
            Hypocalcemia
        Carbon Dioxide (CO_2)
            Hypercapnia
            Hypocapnia
        Chloride (Cl^-)
            Hyperchloremia
            Hypochloremia
        Magnesium (Mg^{++})
            Hypermagnesemia
            Hypomagnesemia
        Potassium (K^+)
            Hyperkalemia
            Hypokalemia
        Phosphate (PO_4)
        Sodium (Na^+)
            Hypernatremia
            Hyponatremia
    Hematology
        Erythrocytes
        Red Blood Cells (RBC)

Hematocrit (Hct)
Hemoglobin (Hgb)
Leukocytes (WBC)
Neutrophils
    Segs and Bands
Lymphocytes
Monocytes
Eosinophils
Basophils
Blood and Serum
    Acetoacetate
    Alkaline Phosphatase
    Alpha$_1$-antitrypsin
    Bicarbonate (HCO_3^-)
    Bilirubin
    Creatine (CPK)
    Creatinine
    Glucose (Fasting)
    Lactic Dehydrogenase
    Pressure of Carbon Dioxide
    pH
    Protein Albumin Globulin
    Blood Urea Nitrogen (BUN)
Urine
    Specific Gravity
    Glucose
    Protein
    Microscopic Exam — Casts
    RBC
    Crystals
Pleural Fluid
    Pleural Transudate
    Pleural Exudate
Cerebrospinal Fluid
Blood Specimen Tubes

ARTERIAL BLOOD GAS

Arterial blood gases provide precise measuren.
acid – base balance of the body. Respiratory and/or n.
dysfunctions may be accurately interpreted with an ai.
blood sample. For accurate interpretation, the patient's to.
clinical status must be considered when obtaining a blood
sample. Care should be taken not to obtain a venous sample,
because venous blood reflects local metabolic rates, and improper treatment may result.

Technique

1. Verify physician order.
2. Collect necessary equipment.
   a. Alcohol or disinfectant
   b. Sterile 3- to 5-ml syringe
   c. Needles (20- to 23-gauge)
   d. 1/1000 sodium heparin
   e. Sterile gauze
   f. Needle stopper or seal
   g. Container for ice bath

Note that most hospitals use blood gas kits that contain
the equipment needed to draw an arterial blood gas sample.
Also, with some patients the therapist may need to use a 1% or
2% Xylocaine solution for local anesthesia. This procedure
requires the injection of Xylocaine subcutaneously (wheal stick)
prior to the initial sample.

3. Fill out proper paper work (varies with each hospital).
4. *Wash hands.*
5. Introduce yourself to the patient and explain the
procedure (in layman's terms).
6. Heparinize the syringe and needle.
7. Position the patient's arm for accessibility.
8. Complete a modified Allen test (for radial site).
9. Prepare site (disinfect).
10. Palpate artery (take your time).
11. Gently insert the needle, with bevel up, into the skin
(the syringe should be held at a 45-degree angle before
insertion).

12. Gently advance the needle until a flash of blood fills e hub of the needle, stop advancement of the needle, and llow for the syringe to fill with 1 to 2 ml of blood.

13. Remove the needle, taking care not to put pressure on the site while removing the needle. The needle could tear underlying tissue.

14. Place pressure on the site after the needle is removed, making sure that the pressure is also applied to an area beyond the site. Due to the angle of the stick, you are puncturing the artery beyond the site. If you use only one finger you could miss applying pressure to the punctured artery.

15. Hold pressure for 5 minutes or longer, until no bleeding is seen. After 5 minutes, rub your finger along the site and feel for any raised areas; if bleeding is seen or raised areas are felt, reapply pressure.

16. Place the blood sample in the ice bath with a needle stopper or seal. By placing the sample in ice you may obtain the proper values.

17. Chart taking of the sample in the patient's records.

Normal Ranges

Normal blood gas ranges are presented in Tables 3–1 through 3–3.

Table 3–1. NORMAL BLOOD GAS RANGES AT SEA LEVEL

Test	Arterial	Mean
pH (units)	7.35–7.45	7.40
Pa_{CO_2} (mmHg)	35–45	40
Pa_{O_2} (mmHg)*	80–100	90
HCO_3^- mEq/L	22–26	24
BE (mEq/L)	±2	0
O_2 (sat%)	95–100	97

*The Pa_{O_2} will change with age.

Table 3–2. NORMAL BLOOD GAS
RANGES ABOVE SEA LEVEL
(5200 FEET)

Test	Arterial	Mean
pH (units)	7.35–7.45	7.40
Pa_{CO_2} (mmHg)	34–38	36
Pa_{O_2} (mmHg)	65–75	70
HCO_3^- mEq/L	22–26	24
BE (mEq/L)	±2	0
O_2 (sat%)	92–94	93

Table 3–3. NORMAL BLOOD GAS
RANGES FOR PREMATURE INFANTS

Test	Arterial	Mean
pH (units)	7.35–7.39	7.37
Pa_{CO_2} (mmHg)	38–44	41
Pa_{O_2} (mmHg)	65–80	72
HCO_3^- mEq/L	22–26	24
BE (mEq/L)	−10 to −2	−6
O_2 (sat%)	40–90	65

Interpretation

Interpretation of blood gases is presented in Tables 3–4
through 3–6.

NORMAL LAB VALUES FOR ELECTROLYTES, HEMATOLOGY, URINE, AND CEREBROSPINAL FLUID

Normal lab values are provided in Table 3–7.

Table 3-4. EVALUATION OF VENTILATORY STATUS AND METABOLIC ACID–BASE STATUS

Classification of Pa$_{CO_2}$

Pa$_{CO_2}$ < 30 mmHg	Alveolar hyperventilation (respiratory alkalosis)
Pa$_{CO_2}$ 30–50 mmHg	Acceptable alveolar ventilation
Pa$_{CO_2}$ > 50 mmHg	Ventilatory failure (respiratory acidosis)

Classification of Ventilatory State in Conjunction with pH

1. Alveolar hyperventilation (Pa$_{CO_2}$ < 30 mmHg)
   a. pH > 7.50   Acute alveolar hyperventilation
   b. pH 7.40–7.50 Chronic alveolar hyperventilation
   c. pH 7.30–7.40 Compensated metabolic acidosis
   d. pH < 7.30   Partly compensated metabolic acidosis
2. Acceptable alveolar ventilation (Pa$_{CO_2}$ 30–50 mmHg)
   a. pH > 7.50   Metabolic alkalosis
   b. pH 7.30–7.50 Acceptable ventilatory and metabolic acid–base status
   c. pH < 7.30   Metabolic acidosis
3. Ventilatory failure (Pa$_{CO_2}$ > 50 mmHg)
   a. pH > 7.50   Partly compensated metabolic alkalosis
   b. pH 7.30–7.50 Chronic ventilatory failure
   c. pH < 7.30   Acute ventilatory failure

(From Shapiro, BA: Clinical Application of Blood Gases, ed 3. Year Book Medical Publishers, Chicago, 1983, with permission.)

Table 3–5. SEVEN PRIMARY BLOOD GAS CLASSIFICATIONS*

Classification	Pa_{CO_2}	pH	$[HCO_3^-]p$	BE
Primary ventilatory				
1. Acute ventilatory failure	↑	↓	N	N
2. Chronic ventilatory failure	↑	N↓	↑	↑
3. Acute alveolar hyperventilation	↓	↑	N	N
4. Chronic alveolar hyperventilation	↓	N	↓	↓
Primary acid–base				
1. Uncompensated acidosis	N	↓	↓	↓
Uncompensated alkalosis	N	↑	↑	↑
2. Partly compensated acidosis	↓	↓	↓	↓
Partly compensated alkalosis	↑	↑	↑	↑
3. Compensated alkalosis or acidosis	↑ or ↓	N	↑ or ↓	↑ or ↓

*Arrows indicate depressed or elevated values; N is normal; and BE is base excess.
(From Shapiro, BA: Clinical Application of Blood Gases, ed 3. Year Book Medical Publishers, Chicago, 1983, with permission.)

Table 3–6. CHANGES IN OXYHEMOGLOBIN DISSOCIATION AS REFLECTED BY SHIFTS OF P_{50}

Right Shifts or Increased P_{50}	Left Shifts or Decreased P_{50}
Due to Increases of 2,3 DPG and P_{50} 7.4	*Due to Decreases of 2,3 DPG and P_{50} 7.4*
Increased inorganic phosphorus (uremia)	Hypophosphatemia
Alkalosis of red cells	Acidosis of red cells
Hypoxia	Hyperbaric oxygenation
Thyroxine excess	Thyroxine deficit
Hexokinase deficiency	Pyruvate kinase deficiency
Anemia	Storage of blood
Increased androgen hormone	
Direct or Unknown Mechanism	*Direct or Unknown Mechanism*
Increased temperature	Decreased temperature
Acidemia (Bohr effect)*	Alkalemia (Bohr effect)*
Young red cells	Decreased red cell Hb concentration
Increased cell Hb concentration	Decreased P_{CO_2}
Erythrocytosis	Decreased anion concentration
Altered Hb† (Kansas, Seattle HbE)	Altered Hb† (carboxy Hb, met Hb, Chesapeake, Rainier, Yakima, Kempry)

*Effect is reduced by temperature and in women according to Boning.

†A complete summary of altered Hb with low and high O_2 P_{50} values was presented by Stomatoyannopoulos and co-workers.

(From Miller, MF: Laboratory Evaluation of Pulmonary Function. JB Lippincott, St. Louis, 1987, p 360, with permission.)

Table 3-7. NORMAL LAB VALUES

Electrolytes	Specimen	Normal Values
Calcium (Ca^{++})	Serum	Adults: 8.5-10.5 mg/dl
		4.3-5.3 mEq/L
Carbon dioxide (CO_2)	Whole blood	Arterial: 19-24 mEq/L
		Venous: 22-26 mEq/L
Chloride (Cl^-)	Serum	95-108 mEq/L
Magnesium (Mg^{++})	Serum	1.8-3.0 mg/dl
		1.5-2.5 mEq/L
Potassium (K^+)	Serum	3.6-5.0 mEq/L
Phosphate (PO_4)	Serum	1.5-4.5 U/dl (Bodansky)
Sodium (Na^+)	Serum	135-148 mEq/L
Hematology		
Red blood cell count		Adult male: 4.5-6.0 million/μL
		Adult female: 4.0-5.5 million/μL
Hemoglobin		Adult male: 14-18 g/dl
		Adult female: 12-16 g/dl
Hematocrit		Adult male: 40%-50%
		Adult female: 37%-47%
White blood cell count		Adults: 4500-11,000/μL
Neutrophils		Adults: 54%-75% (3000-7500/μL)
Band neutrophils		Adults: 3%-8% (150-700/μL)

(continued)

Table 3-7—*Continued*

Hematology	Normal Values
Lymphocytes	Adults: 25%–40% (1500–4500/μL)
Monocytes	Adults: 2%–8% (100–500/μL)
Eosinophils	Adults: 1%–4% (50–400/μL)
Basophils	Adults: 0%–1% (25–100/μL)
Creatine CPK (creatine phosphokinase)	Males: 5–55 mU/ml
	Females: 5–35 mU/ml
Creatinine	0.6–1.5 mg/100 ml
Glucose (fasting)	70–110 mg/100 ml
Lactic dehydrogenase	60–120 U/ml
Pressure of carbon dioxide	Arterial: 35–45 mmHg
	Venous: 40–50 mmHg
pH	Arterial: 7.35–7.45
	Venous: 7.32–7.42
Protein albumin globulin	Total: 6–8 g/100 ml
Blood urea nitrogen (BUN)	8–20 mg/dl

Urine

Specific gravity	1.016–1.040
Glucose	Average, 130 mg/24 hours
Protein quantitatives	<150 mg/24 hours
Sodium	40–180 mEq/24 hours
Uric acids	0.3–0.8 g/24 hours
pH	4.6–8.0
Urine output	800–1200 ml/24 hours

Cerebrospinal Fluid

Appearance	Clear, colorless
Immunoglobulin IgA	0–0.6 mg/dl
Immunoglobulin IgG	0–8.6 mg/dl
Immunoglobulin IgM	0–1.3 mg/dl
pH	7.30–7.40
P_{CO_2}	42–52 mmHg
P_{O_2}	40–44 mmHg

(From Byrne, JC, Saxton, DF, et al: Laboratory Test Implications for Nursing Care, ed 2. Addison-Wesley, Menlo Park, CA, 1986, with permission.)

INCREASES, DECREASES, CAUSES, AND SYMPTOMS OF ALTERED LAB WORK

Please note that normals and units given in this chapter may vary from one institution to another. Also, that the causes and symptoms for increased and decreased values given here are only *possible* causes and symptoms and are not to take the place of a complete history and physical.

Electrolytes

Calcium (Ca^{++})

Normal values:* 8.5 – 10.5 mg/100 ml

Hypercalcemia

Possible causes for increased values: vitamin D intoxication, bony metastases, sarcoidosis, thiazide, adrenal insufficiency; with increased metabolic alkalosis — milk-alkali syndrome; with a decreased BUN — hyperparathyroidism.

Possible symptoms for increased values: *Mild to moderate:* bone pain, pathologic fractures, flank pain from renal stones. *Severe:* intractable nausea, vomiting, dehydration, stupor, coma, cardiac arrest.

Hypocalcemia

Possible causes for decreased lab values: tetany, hypoparathyroidism, vitamin D deficiency, renal failure, alkalosis, steroids, diarrhea; increased gamma globulin — sarcoidosis.

Possible symptoms for decreased lab values: *Mild to moderate:* tingling sensation around the mouth and in the fingertips, abdominal and skeletal muscle cramps. *Severe:* carpopedal spasms and tetany leading to convulsions.

Carbon Dioxide (CO_2)

Normal values: 19 – 24 mEq/L

Hypercapnia

Possible causes for increased values: ventilatory failure (respiratory acidosis) hypoventilation; drugs — aldosterone, bicarbonate, ethacrynic acid, hydrocortisone, laxatives (abuse), metolazone, prednisone, thiazides, tromethamine, and viomycin.

Hypocapnia

Possible causes for decreased values: hyperventilation; drugs — acetazolamide, dimercaprol, dimethadione, methicillin, nitrofurantoin, phenformin, tetracycline, triamterene; with an increase in potassium and chloride — renal tubular acidosis; lactic acidosis; and diabetic ketoacidosis.

Chloride (Cl^-)

Normal values: 95 – 108 mEq/L

Hyperchloremia

Possible causes for increased values: uremia; salt intake; cardiac decompensation; drugs — chlorothiazide (prolonged), corticosteroids, guanethidine, marihuana, phenylbutazone.

Possible symptoms for increased values: overshadowed by symptoms of hypernatremia.

Hypochloremia

Possible causes for decreased values: vomiting, diarrhea, excessive perspiration, COPD, metabolic alkalosis, pneumonia, fever, dehydration, Cushing's syndrome; drugs — aldosterone, bicarbonate, cortisone, diuretics, laxatives.

Possible symptoms for decreased values: overshadowed by symptoms of hyponatremia.

Magnesium (Mg^{++})

Normal values: 1.5 – 2.5 mEq/L

Hypermagnesemia

Possible causes for increased values: uremia, renal insufficiency, parathyroidectomy, antacids.

Possible symptoms for increased values: *Mild to moderate:* reduced nerve and muscle activity, impaired respiration, lethargy. *Severe:* coma, cardiac arrest.

Hypomagnesemia

Possible causes for decreased values: severe malabsorption, alcoholism, diabetic acidosis, renal disease, diarrhea (decreased potassium and increased CO_2 — hypokalemic — chloremic alkalosis).

Possible symptoms for decreased values: *Mild to moderate:* tremors, painful paresthesia, nerve and muscle irritability, increased blood pressure and heart rate. *Severe:* disorientation, convulsions.

Potassium (K^+)

Normal values: 3.5–5.0 mEq/L

Hyperkalemia

Possible causes for increased values: trauma, infection, acute renal failure, can cause arrhythmias, muscle weakness, metabolic acidosis (increases in BUN — Addison's disease); drugs — tetracycline, spironolactone, marihuana, epinephrine.

Possible symptoms for increased values: *Mild to moderate:* irritability, nausea, diarrhea, abdominal cramps, moderate weakness, flaccid paralysis, difficulty in breathing and speaking. *Severe:* ventricular fibrillation, death.

Hypokalemia

Possible causes for decreased values: alkalosis, diarrhea, vomiting, nasogastric suction, diabetic ketoacidosis (with an increased CO_2 — Cushing's syndrome), diuretics, primary and secondary hyperaldosteronism with chronic congestive heart failure, anti-inflammatory drugs.

Possible symptoms for decreased values: *Mild:* malaise, thirst, polyuria. *Moderate:* muscle weakness, decreased reflexes, loss of muscle tone causing cardiac arrhythmias, weak pulse and falling blood pressure, nausea, vomiting, decreased intestinal motility, decreased respiratory functioning. *Severe:* respiratory or cardiac arrest, death.

Phosphate (PO$_4$)

Normal Values: 1.5–4.5 U/dl

Possible causes for increased values: renal insufficiency (with increases in BUN and creatine — chronic glomerular disease) (with a decrease in calcium — hypoparathyroidism); drugs — anabolic steroids, methicillin, phosphates.

Possible causes for decreased values: diabetic ketoacidosis (with increased calcium — hyperparathyroidism) (with an increased calcium and an increased alkaline and phosphate — rickets), renal tubular acidosis, malabsorption syndrome, alkaline antacids, anticonvulsants, epinephrine, insulin, oral contraceptives, phenobarbital.

Sodium (Na$^+$)

Normal values: 135–148 mEq/L

Hypernatremia

Possible causes for increased values: Cushing's syndrome, hyperadrenocorticism (with hyperglycemia, hypothalamic lesions, head trauma), dehydration.

Possible symptoms for increased values: *Mild to moderate:* dry, sticky mucous membranes, intense thirst, flushed skin, agitation, restlessness, and decreased reflexes. *Severe:* hypermania and convulsions.

Hyponatremia

Possible causes for decreased values: (with loss of body fluids — alkali) diuretics, burns, trauma, adrenal insufficiency (with decreased chloride — vomiting, diarrhea, tube drainage) (with increased BUN and creatine — chronic renal insufficiency), paracentesis (with inappropriate ADH syndrome and decreased sodium — bronchogenic carcinoma), pulmonary infections.

Possible symptoms for decreased values: *Mild to moderate:* weakness, confusion, stupor, apprehension, abdominal cramps. *Severe:* hypovolemic shock, death.

Hematology

Erythrocytes

> Normal values: males — 4.5 – 5.5 million/mm³
> females — 4.2 – 5.4 million/mm³

Red Blood Cells (RBC)

Possible causes for increased values: type 1 polycythemia, type 2 polycythemia — COPD, diarrhea, dehydration, cyanotic congenital heart disease with hypoxia (living in high altitudes — hypoxemic hypoxia).

Possible causes for decreased values: hemorrhage, leukemia, decreased production of RBC, myelophthisis, anemia, and Addison's disease.

Hematocrit (Hct)

> Normal values: males — 39% – 54%
> females — 37% – 47%

Possible causes for increased values: dehydration, shock, erythrocytosis, pancreatitis (acute).

Possible causes for decreased values: anemias, acute blood loss, increased fluid intake.

Hemoglobin (Hgb)

> Normal values: males — 14 – 18 g/100 ml
> females — 12 – 16 g/100 ml

Possible causes for increased values: polycythemia, congestive heart failure, COPD, high altitudes, and dehydration.

Possible causes for decreased values: anemia, pregnancy, hemorrhage, increase in fluid intake, iron deficiency, sickle-cell anemia, hemoglobin C disease (folic acid deficiency, vitamin B_{12} deficiency).

Leukocytes (WBC)

> Normal values: total 4500 – 11000/μL

Possible causes for increased values: acute infections, following surgery, trauma, severe sepsis.

Possible causes for decreased values: leukemia, agranulocytosis.

Neutrophils

Normal values: 54% – 75%

Segs and Bands

Possible causes for increased values: bacterial infection, neoplasms, and electroshock therapy; drugs — catecholamines, corticosteroids.

Possible causes for decreased values: familial benign neutropenia, starvation, increased ingestion of alcohol or drugs.

Lymphocytes

Normal values: 20% – 25%

Monocytes

Normal values: 3% – 8%

Possible causes for increased values: chronic infection, chronic lymphocytic leukemia, viral infections.

Possible causes for decreased values: steroid therapy, congestive heart failure, renal failure.

Eosinophils

Normal values: 2% – 5%

Possible causes for increased values: collagen/allergy, parasitic diseases, eosinophilic leukemia.

Possible causes for decreased values: steroid therapy, acute and chronic stress, excess ACTH (cortisone, epinephrine).

Basophils

Normal values: 0 – 1%

Possible causes for increased values: myeloproliferative disease.

Possible causes for decreased values: anaphylactic reaction, steroids, hyperthyroidism, radiation therapy.

Blood and Serum

Acetoacetate

Normal values: 0.3 – 2.0 mg/100 ml
Possible causes for increased values: diabetic ketoacidosis.

Alkaline Phosphatase

Normal Values: adults — 13 – 39 IU/L
                     children and infants — 13 – 104 IU/L
Possible causes for increased values: liver and blood disease, carcinoma with bone metastasis, Paget's disease, Gaucher's disease (with a decrease in calcium — osteomalacia).

Alpha$_1$-antitrypsin

Normal values: 200 – 400 mg/100 ml
Possible causes for increased values: early inflammation, pneumonia, arthritis.
Possible causes for decreased values: COPD, emphysema.

Bicarbonate (HCO$_3^-$)

Normal values: 22 – 26 mEq/L
Possible causes for increased values: metabolic alkalosis, chronic respiratory acidosis, the drugs aldosterone and viomycin.
Possible causes for decreased values: metabolic acidosis, chronic respiratory alkalosis, triamterene, dehydration.

Bilirubin

Normal values: total 0.1 – 1.0 mg/100 ml

Possible causes for increased values: hemolytic anemia, hepatitis, biliary obstruction, hemolytic disease of the newborn, direct or with abnormal albumin, globulin and enzymes, liver disease, acute alcoholic hepatitis, carcinoma of the head of the pancreas.

Possible causes for decreased values: pernicious anemia, drugs—barbiturates, corticosteroids, thioridazine, sulfonamides.

Creatine (CPK)

Normal values: males—5–55 mU/ml
females—5–35 mU/ml

Possible causes for increased values: muscle damage, myocardial infarction, muscle disease, polymyositis, cerebral infarct, Duchenne's dystrophy, cardiac surgery, rejection of heart transplant, hepatic coma, severe alcohol intoxication.

Creatinine

Normal values: 0.6–1.5 mg/100 ml
Possible causes for increased values: nephritis, renal insufficiency, urinary tract obstruction, with increased BUN—congestive heart failure.

Glucose (Fasting)

Normal values: 70–110 mg/100 ml
Possible causes for increased values: drugs, steroids, diabetes mellitus, infections, uremia, stress (with decreased cholesterolemia—hyperthyroidism), pancreatic insufficiency (with hypernatremia—hyperglycemia).

Possible causes for decreased values: insulin, aspirin, ascorbic acid, pituitary hypofunction (with increased BUN—Addison's disease), liver disease, hypoglycemia.

Lactic Dehydrogenase

Normal values: 60–120 U/ml

Possible causes for increased values: hypoxia, increased muscular activity, congestive heart failure, hemorrhage, shock, pulmonary embolism, myocardial infarction, pernicious anemia, viral hepatitis, pneumonia, renal infarcts.

Pressure of Carbon Dioxide

Normal values: arterial — 35 – 45 mmHg
venous — 40 – 50 mmHg

Possible causes for increased values: respiratory acidosis, metabolic alkalosis (hypokalemic — chloremic), alkalosis with decreased potassium and decreased chloride.

Possible causes for decreased values: respiratory alkalosis, metabolic acidosis, uremic acidosis, diabetic ketoacidosis, lactic acidosis (with increased chloride and decreased potassium — renal tubular acidosis).

pH

Normal values: arterial — 7.35 – 7.45
venous — 7.32 – 7.42

Possible causes for increased values: hypocapnia, vomiting, fever (increased CO_2 — metabolic alkalosis) (alkali — overmedicated), Cushing's disease, diarrhea, high altitude, hyperventilation, hysteria, peptic ulcer therapy, renal disorders, salicylate intoxication.

Possible causes for decreased values: hypercapnia, uremia, diabetic acidosis, hemorrhage, nephritis, Addison's disease, emphysema, hepatic dysfunction, hypoventilation, pneumonia, respiratory acidosis.

Protein Albumin Globulin

Normal values: total 6 – 8.4 g/100 ml

Possible causes for increased values: shock (with high globulin and normal or low albumin — multiple myeloma, macroglobulinemia, sarcoidosis) (with high albumin and high globulin — dehydration).

Possible causes for decreased values: malnutrition, leukemia, nephrosis, hemorrhage (with low albumin — renal disease and ulcerative colitis) (with low albumin and low globulin — severe burns, near drowning, and scleroderma).

Blood Urea Nitrogen (BUN)

Normal values: 8 – 20 mg/100 ml

Possible causes for increased values: renal insufficiency, nitrogen metabolism, gastrointestinal bleeding, decreased renal flow, shock, congestive heart failure, glomerular nephritis, pyelonephritis, sepsis, fever (dehydration — caused by burns, profuse diarrhea, vomiting, excessive perspiration).

Possible causes for decreased values: hepatic failure, nephrosis, pregnancy, amyloidosis, cirrhosis, low-protein diet, malnutrition, hemodialysis.

Urine

Specific Gravity

Normal values: 1.016 – 1.040

Possible causes for increased values: congestive heart failure, fever, vomiting, diabetes mellitus, intravenous albumin, liver disorders, x-ray contrast media.

Possible causes for decreased values: (decreased K^+, Ca^{++}, with increased Cl^- — distal renal tubular disease and chronic renal disease), (with increased Ca^{++} and decreased K^+ — hypokalemic and hypercalcemic nephropathy), hypothermia (sarcoidosis, bone disease, hyperparathyroidism — with hypercalcemia).

Glucose

Normal values: average negative

Possible causes for increased values: (glycosuria with increased blood glucose — diabetes mellitus; glycosuria with decreased blood glucose — low renal threshold for glucose resorption), drugs — aspirin, ammonium chloride, corticosteroids, ephedrine; meningitis, cerebrovascular accident, Cushing's disease, Fanconi's syndrome, infection, intracranial injury, pancreatitis, pregnancy.

Decreased or negative values are normal.

Protein

Normal values: quantitative — 2 – 8 mg/dl or 40 – 80 mg/24 hours

Possible causes for increased values: renal glomerular disease, multiple myeloma, lymphoma, amyloidosis.

Decreased or negative values are normal.

Microscopic Exam — Casts

Normal values: negative

Possible causes for the appearance of casts: WBC casts — pyelonephritis; RBC casts — acute glomerulonephritis; hyaline casts with proteinuria — nephrotic syndrome; shock.

RBC

Normal values: negative

Possible causes for increased values: hematuria — hemorrhagic cystitis or calculi in the renal pelvis, tuberculosis, tumors of the renal collecting tubular system.

Crystals

Normal values: negative

Possible causes for increased values: (with amorphous substance and increased uric acid — possible gouty nephropathy; calcium oxalate crystals with increase serum calcium — suggest hypercalcemia) leukemia, theophylline therapy.

Pleural Fluid

Pleural Transudate

Possible causes: any factors that would cause increased

Table 3-8. CEREBROSPINAL FLUID

Appearance	Causes
Normal to slightly turbid	With 10–60 neutrophils, glucose slightly decreased, protein normal to moderately increased — brain abscess.
Normal	With 50–100 lymphocytes, glucose slightly decreased, with slight increase in protein — encephalitis.
Red, cloudy, xanthochromic	With many RBC, glucose normal, protein markedly increased — subarachnoid hemorrhage.
Xanthochromic to normal	With 10–60 lymphocytes, normal glucose, protein normal to a slight increase — subdural hemorrhage.
Turbid to purulent	With greater than 1000 neutrophils, glucose is decreased, protein is greatly increased — acute pyogenic meningitis.
Normal to slightly turbid	With 10–60 lymphocytes, glucose slightly decreased, protein slightly increased — aseptic meningitis.
Normal to hazy	With 10–60 lymphocytes, glucose decreased, protein slightly increased — fungal meningitis.
Slightly turbid	With 50–100 lymphocytes, glucose decreased, protein moderately increased — tuberculous meningitis.
Normal	With 100–500 lymphocytes, glucose normal, protein slightly increased — viral meningitis.
Normal	With 10–60 lymphocytes, glucose normal, protein slightly increased — multiple sclerosis.

venous pressure or decreased plasma albumin, congestive heart failure, hepatic cirrhosis, or hypoproteinemia resulting from nephrotic syndrome.

Pleural Exudate

Effusion caused by damage to mesothelial lining of the pleural cavity — pneumonia, tuberculosis, neoplasms, trauma, rheumatoid disease, pulmonary infarct.

Possible causes of increase in pleural fluid volumes: bacterial pneumonia, bronchogenic carcinoma, congestive heart failure, hypoproteinemia, liver disease, lymphoma, metastatic carcinoma, neoplasms, nephrotic syndrome, pulmonary infarcts, rheumatoid disease, systemic lupus erythematosus, trauma, tuberculosis, viral pneumonia.

Cerebrospinal Fluid

This is presented in Table 3–8.

BLOOD SPECIMEN TUBES

These are presented in Tables 3–9 and 3–10.

Table 3–9. BLOOD SPECIMEN TUBE REQUIREMENTS

Color of Tube Top	Tube Contents
Black	Sodium oxalate
Blue	Sodium citrate
Brown	Minimal lead content
Gray	Glycolytic inhibitor
Green	Heparin
Lavendar	EDTA
Red	No additives
Yellow	No additives (sterile)

Table 3-10. COLOR TUBES
AND THEIR RELATED LABS

Red Top
Ethanol, salicylates, BUN, electrolytes, Monospot, serum protein, electrophoresis, phenobarbital, phenytoin, theophylline, procainamide, gentamicin, tobramycin, lithium, bromide, alcohol (site cannot be cleaned with alcohol), calcium, amylase, acetone, protein, albumin, bilirubin, IgG, IgA, IgM, and LD isoenzymes.

Purple Top
CBC, Hgb and Hct, WBC, platelets, and most other hematology (Note that carbon monoxide and methemoglobin are also collected in purple top tubes.)

Blue Top
G-6-PD assay, PT, APTT, thrombin time, fibrinogen, and most other coagulation labs

Gray Top
Glucose

Green Top
Ammonia, lactic acid (These should be placed in ice.)

BIBLIOGRAPHY

The works listed below are also suggested readings that will give the reader more information concerning the chapter content.

Byrne, CJ: Laboratory Tests. Addison-Wesley, Menlo Park, CA, 1986.

Shapiro, BA: Clinical Application of Blood Gases, ed 3. Year Book Medical Publishers, Chicago, 1982.

Spearman, CB: Egan's Fundamentals of Respiratory Therapy. CV Mosby, St. Louis, 1982.

Widmann, FK: Clinical Interpretation of Laboratory Tests, ed 9. FA Davis, Philadelphia, 1983.

NOTES

4 Respiratory Pathophysiology

PULMONARY INSUFFICIENCY

Degree of respiratory failure that may occur when the exchange of respiratory gases between the circulating blood and the ambient atmosphere is impaired. This impairment can be caused by disease or trauma that to some degree anatomically alters the lung and chest wall.

Clinical information may be gained by inspecting the chest. The majority of this information should be gathered without the patient's knowledge. This is done by listening and by observation of the patient.

Things to Look For

Is the patient short of breath while talking? Note the use of accessory muscles and retractions. Note the patient's posture, respiratory rate and pattern, pursed-lip breathing, grunting, or nasal flaring. Also note symmetry of the chest, skin color, nailbeds, digital clubbing, type of cough (dry, hacking, loose, wet). Is the cough productive, and if it is, how much? When is the cough present (morning, night, all the time)? What time of the year is the cough present? Note the color of the sputum, audible wheezing or rhonchi, evidence of edema or dehydration.

This information is the basis for proper treatment of the patient with respiratory problems.

ANXIETY ASSESSMENT FINDINGS

The patient's fear of being in a hospital or physician's office or just the fear of the unknown can affect your physical findings of the patient. The appearance, conversation, behavior, and vital signs may dramatically increase when anxiety is present. A thorough patient interview and physical examination are necessary for prompt and proper treatment. Help reduce the amount of anxiety by asking open-ended questions. When needed, obtain additional information from the patient's family, if possible.

The following are things to look for in patients with anxiety[*]:

Appearance — muscular tension, pale clammy skin, fatigue, and restlessness.

Conversation — does the patient frequently ask questions? Shifts topic of conversation, describes fears with a sense of helplessness, and avoids focusing on his own feelings?

---

[*]Though most of the symptoms listed may be caused by factors other than anxiety, a thorough physical examination with proper lab work can give you a good overall clinical picture.

Behavior—does the patient have a shortened attention span? Does the patient have an inability to follow directions?

Physiologic signs—increased heart rate, respiratory rate, blood pressure, and perspiration.

RESPIRATORY BREATHING PATTERNS

Eupnea

Normal respiratory rate and rhythm with occasional deep breath.

Tachypnea

Increased respiratory rate as seen in patients with fever, pneumonia, respiratory insufficiency, lesions of the brain's respiratory control center.

Bradypnea

Slower respiratory rate but regular, affected by narcotics, tumors, alcohol, and during normal sleep.

Apnea

Absence of breathing, which may be periodic.

Hyperpnea

Deeper than normal breaths but with a normal rate.

Cheyne-Stokes

Slower respiratory rate that gets faster and deeper than normal, with periods of apnea of 20 to 60 seconds.

Causes are increased intracranial pressure, severe congestive heart failure, meningitis, and drug overdose.

Biot's

Faster and deeper respiratory rate with abrupt pauses between breaths. Each breath has the same depth.

Causes are spinal meningitis or other central nervous system conditions.

Kussmaul's

Faster and deeper than normal respiratory rate without pauses. Breathing sounds are labored, with deep breaths that resemble sighs.

Causes may be renal failure or diabetic ketoacidosis.

Apneustic

Prolonged gasping inspiration, followed by short, inefficient expiration. It can be caused by lesions in the respiratory control center.

LOCATIONS FOR PLACEMENT OF THE STETHOSCOPE

Figures 4–1 and 4–2 show the frontal and dorsal placement of the stethoscope.

BREATH SOUNDS

Abnormal

The results of a movement by pulmonary physicians five years ago to change terms such as rales, sibilant, musical, and so on to more descriptive terms have made breath sounds easier to describe and easier to explain.

Recommended Terms	Terms Used Before 1982
Crackles	Rales or crepitation
Wheezes	Sibilant rales, musical rales, and sibilant rhonchus
Rhonchi	Low-pitched wheeze and sonorous rales
Stridor	Stridor (no change)

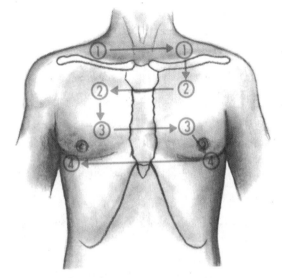

Figure 4–1. Stethoscope placement: frontal. Note that the locations for placement of the stethoscope are the same general locations for percussion. (From Bates, B: A Guide to Physical Examination, ed 3. JB Lippincott, Philadelphia, 1983, p 138, with permission.)

Normal

Vesicular breath sounds are heard over most of the chest, except over major airways. The pitch is low in tone. The inspiratory-to-expiratory ratio is 1 : 3. The sound is said to be breezy.

Tracheal breath sounds are heard over the trachea. The pitch is very high in tone. The inspiratory-to-expiratory ratio is 5 : 6. The sound is said to be loud, harsh, and tubular.

Bronchial breath sounds are heard over the major central airways. They are high in pitch, with an inspiratory-to-expiratory ratio of 2 : 3, and are described as hollow or tubular in sound.

Bronchial-vesicular breath sounds are heard over the

major central airways. The pitch is of medium tone, with an inspiratory-to-expiratory ratio of 1 : 1, and the sound is breezy.

CLASSIFICATION OF DYSPNEA

Class I — dyspnea only on severe exertion (appropriate).

Class II — can keep pace with persons of the same age and body size on level surface without breathlessness, but not on hills or stairs.

Class III — can walk a mile at own pace without dyspnea but cannot keep pace on level surface with a normal person.

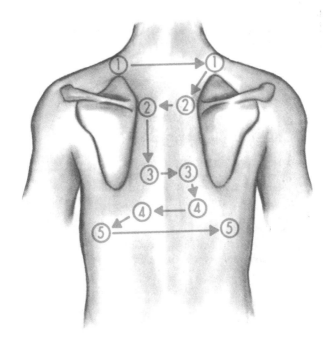

Figure 4 – 2. Stethoscope placement: dorsal. (From Bates, B: A Guide to Physical Examination, ed 3. JB Lippincott, Philadelphia, 1983, p 146, with permission.)

Class IV — dyspnea present after walking about 100 yards on a level surface with a normal person or on climbing one flight of stairs.

Class V — dyspnea on even less activity or even at rest.

EXAMINATION OF THE TRACHEA

With certain pulmonary conditions the trachea may shift toward or away from the affected lung. Some causes that would pull the trachea toward the affected side are pulmonary atelectasis, pulmonary fibrosis, pneumonectomy, and diaphragmatic paralysis. When the trachea is pushed to the unaffected side, the possible causes are neck tumors, thyroid enlargement, mediastinal mass, massive pleural effusion, tension pneumothorax, and hemothorax.

SPUTUM OBSERVATION

This is presented in Table 4–1.

CHEST X-RAYS

Reasons for Obtaining

There are five major reasons for obtaining a chest x-ray:

1. Detect changes in the lung caused by pathologic processes.

2. Determine appropriate therapy.

3. Evaluate effectiveness of treatment.

4. Determine proper tube and catheter placement.

5. Provide a way of trending the progression or decline of lung disease and tumors.

Standard Views

The standard views of the chest are the posteroanterior (P-A) and the lateral view (Figs. 4–3 and 4–4). The *P-A view is preferred* because, since the heart is in the anterior half of the chest, there will be less cardiac magnification. The left

Table 4-1. SPUTUM OBSERVATION

Appearance	Possible Causes
Mucoid, clear, thin, frothy	Bronchial asthma, Legionnaires' disease, pulmonary tuberculosis, emphysema, early chronic bronchitis
Mucopurulent, yellow-green	All of the above and infection, pneumonia, cystic fibrosis
Purulent, yellow, thick, viscid	Bronchiectasis, advanced chronic bronchitis, *Pseudomonas* pneumonia
Apple green, thick pink, thin blood-streaked	*Hemophilus influenzae* pneumonia, streptococcal pneumonia, staphylococcal pneumonia
Blood-rust	*Klebsiella* pneumonia, pneumococcal pneumonia, lung abscess, bronchiectasis, anaerobic infections, aspiration
Black	Smoke, coal dust
Frothy pink	Pulmonary edema
Blood	Pulmonary emboli with infarction, tuberculosis, abscess, trauma, mitral valve disease

lateral view is also preferred because there is less cardiac magnification and a sharper view of the left lower lobe, which is partially obscured on the P-A film.

Correlation Between X-Ray Findings and Physical Examination

There should be a correlation between what is seen on an x-ray and the physical examination. The following is a list of physical findings with related x-ray findings for certain disease states.

Atelectasis

Physical Findings. Elevated diaphragm on the affected side on palpation of the lower chest. Decreased or absent

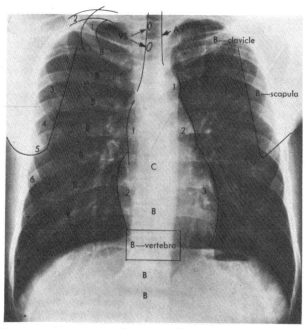

Figure 4-3. Normal chest x-ray. *A*, Air seen in the upper airways. *B*, Bones and ribs have been numbered on the outside of the right thorax; *VS* are the vertebral spinous processes, which should line up and down the middle of the chest; if they don't, the patient should be rotated. If the rotation is great, a new x-ray should be taken. (From Spearman, CB and Sheldon, RL: Egan's Fundamentals of Respiratory Therapy, ed 4. CV Mosby, St. Louis, 1982, p 312, with permission.)

breath sounds on the affected side by auscultation. Shift of the trachea to the affected side only if a large area of the lung is affected.

X-Ray Findings. Shift of the fissure lines and hilar structures toward the affected area and overall loss of volume with elevation of the hemidiaphragm.

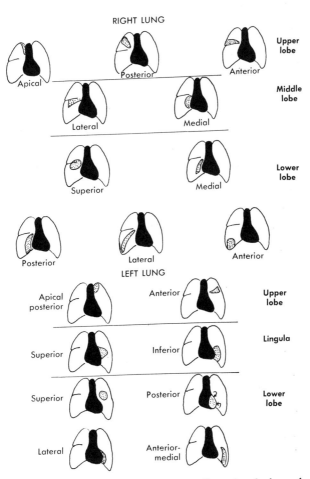

Figure 4–4. Approximate location of infiltrates used when referring to a chest film. (From Spearman, CB and Sheldon, RL: Egan's Fundamentals of Respiratory Therapy, ed 4. CV Mosby, St. Louis, 1982, p 329, with permission.)

Consolidation

Physical Findings. Dullness on percussion over affected areas. Auscultation reveals crackles over the affected area. Whispered voice sounds are usually louder than normal.

X-Ray Findings. Minimal loss of volume with lobar distribution and homogeneous density (whiter area) late in the consolidation process.

Congestive Heart Failure

Physical Findings. Increased heart rate with either a regular or irregular rhythm. A third heart sound (S_3) is a consistent finding. The peripheral pulse may be strong, alternating to a weak pulse every other beat. Pedal edema is usually present during the day but is somewhat relieved after a night of sleep. Patient usually complains of coughing, attacks of severe shortness of breath, fatigue, and weakness.

X-Ray Findings. Usually shows prominent pulmonary blood vessels. Development of Kerley B lines, which are seen in the right base. These Kerley B lines are horizontal and start at the periphery; they are usually 1 mm thick and 1 to 2 cm in length.

Hyperinflation (COPD)

Physical Findings. Barrel chested with decreased breath sounds, wheezing, limited motion of the diaphragm, increased respiratory rate, and the use of accessory muscles to breathe.

X-Ray Findings. Increased A-P chest dimensions and anterior air space. Depressed diaphragms, marked hyperinflation with large lung volumes, and small narrow heart with enlarged intercostal spaces.

Interstitial Fibrosis

Physical Findings. May have a dry, nonproductive cough, dyspnea on exertion, and a history of exposure to inhaled agents.

X-Ray Findings. Peripheral markings are enlarged and white in color. The air-filled airways are seen as clear with dark straight shadows. The peripheral white markings are said to have the appearance of ground glass, representing affected alveolar spaces.

Pleural Effusion

Physical Findings. Decreased breath sounds over affected side, pain on inspiration, coughing, and shortness of breath.

X-Ray Findings. Large volumes of complete "white-out" on the affected side completely obscuring the hemi-diaphragm. With small-volume effusion, only partial "white-out" on the affected side is seen, with only partial obstruction of the hemidiaphragm.

Pneumothorax

Physical Findings. Reduction in movement of the chest wall with decreased breath sounds on the affected side. Heart rate and respiratory rate are increased. The trachea is shifted toward the unaffected side.

X-Ray Findings. Show a pleural line that runs down the chest wall. The trachea is shifted toward the unaffected side.

RESPIRATORY DISEASES

The following is a listing of possible causes, clinical findings, and treatment of common respiratory diseases.

Chronic Bronchitis

Meaning

Chronic inflammation and swelling of the peripheral airway. Excessive mucus production and accumulation. Bronchial airway obstruction. Hyperinflated alveoli.

ͻssible Causes

Exact causes are not known; cigarette smoking, atmospheric pollutants, and repeated infection of the respiratory tract have been linked to the disorder.

Clinical Findings

Pulmonary function tests: decreases in FEF_{25-75}, FEV_1, MVV, PEFR, V_C, IRV; increases in Vt, RV, FRC, VC, FVC.

Chest x-ray: translucent, depressed or flattened diaphragm, spike-like projections on bronchogram, enlarged heart, pulmonary vascular engorgement, and increased anteroposterior chest diameter (barrel chest).

Respiratory Findings

Use of accessory muscles, diminished breath sounds with wheezing and/or rhonchi, chronic cough with excessive sputum production for 3 months per year for two or more successive years.

Arterial Blood Gases

Early — decreased Pa_{O_2}, normal or decreased Pa_{CO_2}, normal or decreased pH.

Advanced Stage — decreased Pa_{O_2}, increased Pa_{CO_2}, increased HCO_3^-, normal or decreased pH.

Treatment

Avoidance of smoking, inhaling of irritants, and infections, mostly people with contagious respiratory tract infections. Mobilize bronchial secretions by nebulizer or aerosol therapy, increased fluid intake, chest physical therapy, postural drainage, deep breathing aids (incentive spirometer), and suctioning. Sympathomimetics (Bronkosol, Alupent, etc.), methylxanthines (aminophylline, etc.), expectorants (Robitussin, etc.), antibiotics (ampicillin, tetracycline). Proper education and psychological and sociologic support.

Emphysema

Meaning

Permanent enlargement and deterioration of air spaces distal to the terminal bronchioles. Destruction of pulmonary capillaries. Weakening of the distal airways, primarily the respiratory bronchioles. Air-trapping.

Types

There are three types of emphysema:
Centrilobular — changes mostly in the respiratory bronchioles.
Panlobular — changes at the alveolar level.
Bullous — changes at the alveolar and respiratory bronchioles.

Possible Causes

Cigarette smoking, alpha$_1$-antitrypsin deficiency, infections of the respiratory tract during childhood, inhaled irritants (sulfur dioxide, nitrogen oxides, and ozone).

Clinical Findings

Pulmonary function tests: increased Vt, RV, FRC, VC; decreased IRV, ERV, FVC, FEF$_{25-75}$, FEV$_1$, MVV, PEFR.
Chest x-ray: increased anteroposterior chest diameter (barrel chest); translucent, depressed, or flattened diaphragm; elongated cardiac silhouette, and small heart.

Respiratory Findings

Increases in respiratory infections, respiratory rate, heart rate, cardiac output, and blood pressure. The patient will show an increase in use of accessory muscles with pursed-lip breathing. Cyanosis and digital clubbing may also be seen.

Arterial Blood Gases

Early stages — decreased Pa$_{O_2}$, normal or decreased Pa$_{CO_2}$, normal or decreased HCO$_3^-$, normal or increased pH.

Advanced stages — decreased Pa_{O_2}, increased Pa_{CO_2}, increased HCO_3^-, normal or decreased pH.

Treatment

Avoidance of smoking, people with contagious respiratory tract infections, and inhaling irritants. Proper nutrition; meals (possible high protein) should be given in small amounts but more often, 6 to 8 a day. Mobilization of bronchial secretions by aerosol or nebulizer therapy, increase in fluids, chest physical therapy, deep breathing aids (incentive spirometer), and suctioning. Supplemental oxygen at low flow. Possible medications —sympathomimetic agents (Bronkosol, Alupent, etc.), methylxanthines (aminophylline), expectorants (Nortussin, Robitussin, etc.), antibiotics, digitalis (Lanoxin, etc.) for patients with ventricular heart failure with emphysema. Proper education of patient and family.

Asthma

Meaning

Smooth muscle constriction of bronchial airways. Excessive production of thick, tenacious tracheobronchial secretions. Hyperinflation of alveoli. Thickening of subepithelial membranes.

Possible Causes

Extrinsic asthma (allergic reaction to pollen, house dust, feathers, etc.). Hypersensitivity to common environmental allergens. Intrinsic asthma (nonallergic or nonatopic), infection, cold air, vapor, drugs (aspirin), emotional stress, and exercise.

Clinical Findings

Pulmonary function tests: decreases in FEF_{25-75}, FEV, MVV, PEFR, VC, IRV, ERV; increases in RV, FRC, RV/TLC ratio.

Chest x-ray: increased anteroposterior chest diameter, translucent, depressed, or flattened diaphragm.

Respiratory Findings

Increased respiratory rate, heart rate, blood pressure, use of accessory muscles, pursed-lip breathing, cough with expectoration, decreased breath sounds with wheezing and/or rhonchi often audible without a stethoscope, and a prolonged expiratory time.

Arterial Blood Gases

Acute — decreased Pa_{O_2}, decreased Pa_{CO_2}, decreased HCO_3^-, increased pH.

Status asthmaticus — decreased Pa_{O_2}, increased Pa_{CO_2}, increased HCO_3^-, decreased pH.

Treatment

Medications: sympathomimetic agents, methylxanthines, corticosteroids. Supplemental oxygen and possible mechanical ventilation in patients with status asthmaticus. Pneumothorax frequently develops in status asthmaticus, necessitating the need for chest tubes. Mobilization of bronchial secretions: suctioning, aerosol therapy, increased fluid intake — systemic, possible chest physical therapy. Environmental control, monitoring arterial blood gases, proper education of the patient, psychological and sociologic support.

Pneumonia

Meaning

Inflammation of the alveoli. Alveolar consolidation.

Possible Causes

Gram-positive, gram-negative organisms, viral, rickettsial infection, psittacosis, varicella, rubella, and aspiration.

Clinical Findings

Pulmonary function tests: decreases in VC, RV, FRC, TLC, Vt.
Chest x-ray: increased opacity (whiter in appearance), increased lung density.

Respiratory Findings

Increases in respiratory rate, heart rate, blood pressure, cough with expectoration, chest pain with decreased chest expansion, bronchial breath sounds with rales/rhonchi/wheezing, possible pleural friction rub.

Arterial Blood Gases

Early stages—decreased Pa_{O_2}, normal to decreased Pa_{CO_2}, normal to decreased HCO_3^-, increased pH.
Advanced stages—decreased Pa_{O_2}, increased Pa_{CO_2}, increased HCO_3^-, decreased pH.

Treatment

Medications: antibiotic agents, sympathomimetic, nonsedative analgesic agents. Oxygen therapy (keeping the Pa_{O_2} 60 to 80 mmHg), possible mechanical ventilation for patients with chronic lung problems and pneumonia, increases in fluid intake, deep breathing aids (IPPB, incentive spirometer), chest physical therapy, nebulizer therapy, possible thoracentesis, bronchoscope, control of fever and excess cough. Keep a close watch for complications.

Pulmonary Edema

Meaning

Interstitial edema, including fluid engorgement of the perivascular and peribronchial spaces and the alveolar wall interstitium, increased surface tension, alveolar shrinkage, frothy secretions throughout the tracheobronchial tree.

Possible Causes

Cardiogenic causes: increases in hydrostatic pressure, arrhythmias, excessive fluid administration, left ventricle failure, mitral valve disease, myocardial infarction, pulmonary embolus, renal failure, systemic hypertension.

Noncardiogenic causes: pulmonary edema, alveolar hypoxia, adult respiratory distress syndrome (ARDS), inhalation of toxic gas (chlorine, sulfur dioxide, ammonia), therapeutic radiation of the lungs, lymphatic insufficiency, overtransfusion or rapid transfusion, uremia, hypoproteinemia, acute nephritis, allergic reaction to drugs, aspiration, central nervous system stimulation, encephalitis, head trauma.

Clinical Findings

Pulmonary function tests: decreases in VC, RV, FRC, TLC, Vt.

Chest x-ray: increased opacity, enlarged heart, prominent pulmonary vessels, Kerley B lines.

Respiratory Findings

Increased respiratory rate, nocturnal dyspnea, cough with expectoration, cyanosis, breath sounds, rales/rhonchi/wheezing, increase in pulmonary wedge pressure — cardiogenic only.

Arterial Blood Gases

Early — decreased Pa_{O_2}, normal or decreased Pa_{CO_2}, normal or decreased HCO_3^-, normal to decreased pH.

Advanced stage — decreased Pa_{O_2}, increased Pa_{CO_2}, increased HCO_3^-, decreased pH.

Pulmonary wedge pressure for cardiogenic pulmonary edema > 12 mmHg.

Treatment

Medications — morphine sulfate, diuretic agents, digitalis, sympathomimetic agents, albumin, possible inhaled ethanol;

ing patients in Fowler's position; hyperinflation and
(keeping Pa_{O_2} 60–80 mmHg); possible intubation with
he-cycled ventilator with PEEP or CPAP. Hemoglobin
w 10 g should be corrected by blood transfusion, fluid
nagement.

Pulmonary Embolism

Meaning

Blockage of the pulmonary vascular system. Pulmonary
infarction. Pulmonary tissue necrosis.

Possible Causes

Prolonged bed rest and/or immobilization; prolonged sitting (car, plane, bus, etc.); congestive heart failure; varicose
veins; long bone fractures — trauma; injury of the soft tissues,
vessels; extensive hip, abdominal, or chest surgery; oral contraceptives; obesity; pregnancy; and burns.

Clinical Findings

Physical Findings: chest pain, increased respiratory rate,
cough with hemoptysis, syncope, lightheadedness, confusion,
cyanosis, breath sounds — rales/rhonchi/wheezing/pleural
friction rub, abnormal perfusion lung scan, pulmonary hypertension, systemic hypotension. ECG — sinus tachycardia or
atrial arrhythmia or possible incomplete right bundle-branch
block.

Arterial Blood Gases

Decreased Pa_{O_2}, normal to decreased Pa_{CO_2}, normal to
decreased HCO_3^-, normal to increased pH.

Treatment

Heparin, dicumarol, supplemental oxygen, possible embo-
lectomy, and treat any cardiac problems that might arise.

Adult Respiratory Distress Syndrome (ARDS)

Meaning

Interstitial and intra-alveolar edema and hemorrhage. Alveolar consolidation. Intra-alveolar hyaline membrane. Pulmonary surfactant deficiency or abnormality. Atelectasis.

Possible Causes

Aspiration; central nervous system disease; cardiopulmonary bypass; congestive heart failure; disseminated intravascular coagulation (DIC); drug overdose; fat or air emboli; fluid overload; infections; inhalation of chlorine, nitrogen dioxide, smoke, or ozone; immunologic reaction.

Clinical Findings

Pulmonary function tests: decreases in VC, RV, FRC, TLC, Vt.

Chest x-ray: increased opacity, diffused alveolar infiltrates (honeycomb effect).

Respiratory Findings

Increased respiratory rate and blood pressure, intercostal retractions, cough, nausea, vomiting, fever, decreased compliance, breath sounds, rales/rhonchi, mental disorientation.

Arterial Blood Gases

Decreased Pa_{O_2}, decreased Pa_{CO_2}, increased pH. These changes occur in the early stages.

Treatment

Medications — diuretic agents, corticosteroids, antibiotic. Hyperinflation and oxygenation. Possible intubation with ventilation and PEEP therapy maintaining $Pa_{O_2} > 60$ mmHg. Possible fluid therapy, watching input and output.

Flail Chest

Meaning and Structural Changes

Double fracture of multiple adjacent ribs. Rib instability. Lung restriction. Atelectasis. Lung collapse.

Possible Causes

Direct compression by a heavy object (automobile or industrial accident).

Clinical Findings

Pulmonary function tests: decreases in VC, RV, FRC, TLC, Vt.

Chest x-ray: rib fractures involving three or more adjacent ribs, or multiple fractures of two or more ribs will increase opacity.

Respiratory Findings

Increased respiratory rate, heart rate, blood pressure; paradoxical chest movement (uneven movement).

Arterial Blood Gases

Early stages—decreased Pa_{O_2}, normal or decreased Pa_{CO_2}, normal or decreased HCO_3^-, normal or increased pH.

Advanced stages—decreased Pa_{O_2}, increased Pa_{CO_2}, increased HCO_3^-, decreased pH.

Treatment

Deep-breathing aids (incentive spirometer), medication for pain, bronchial hygiene, stabilization of fractures, possible mechanical ventilation with PEEP. Look for possible pneumothorax.

Pneumothorax

Meaning or Structural Changes

Lung collapse. Atelectasis. Compression of the great veins and decreased venous return.

Possible Causes

Traumatic pneumothorax (penetrating wounds, also called sucking chest wound). Spontaneous pneumothorax (suddenly without any obvious underlying cause). Iatrogenic pneumothorax (occurs during specific diagnostic or therapeutic procedures).

Clinical Findings

Pulmonary function tests: decreases in VC, RV, FRC, TLC, Vt.
Chest x-ray: localized hyperlucency (PA and lateral view).

Respiratory Findings

Increased difficulty in ventilating if on mechanical ventilator, vital signs will deteriorate, breath sounds will be absent on the affected side, trachea and mediastinum may shift toward unaffected side, possible pleuritic pain, and dry hacking cough.

Treatment

Decompression of the thorax by chest tube insertion or needle aspiration for pneumothorax > 20%, bed rest for pneumothorax < 20%, oxygen therapy, watch for atelectasis — if present deep-breathing aids (incentive spirometer). *IPPB should be given only if the pneumothorax has been corrected or treated.*

Respiratory Care and Surgery

Preoperative Evaluation

History. Chronic cough, shortness of breath, chest pain, smoking, edema in hands and feet, age, previous or existing heart disease, obesity, any chronic disease or muscle weakness noted.

Physical Examination. State of nutrition, movement of the chest wall and abdomen, pursed-lip breathing, rib cage deformities, auscultation of the lungs.

Investigations. Chest x-ray, pulmonary function test, and arterial blood gases.

Management. For heavy smokers, urge them to stop or at least cut down. Patients who are overweight should be placed on a diet — this only for elective surgery. Recent changes in sputum production or color — patients should be placed on antibiotics. Bronchospasm should be treated with bronchodilator drugs. Hypoxemia should be corrected if possible. Avoid excessive premedications. If high risk for pulmonary complication, determine arterial blood gases, at least bedside pulmonary function tests, baseline ECG, and vital signs.

Acute Ventilatory Failure

Meaning

Any cause that would affect ventilation.

Possible Causes

Has many etiologies. You must identify the underlying causes:

Depression of the central drive caused by drug poisoning or craniocerebral trauma

Upper airway obstruction caused by tumors, hemorrhage, or foreign body

Lower airway and parenchymal defects caused by chronic bronchitis, emphysema, asthma, or pulmonary edema

Chest wall disorders caused by kyphoscoliosis, obesity, or birth defects

Neuromuscular defects caused by myasthenia gravis, Guillain Barré syndrome, and respiratory muscle fatigue

Physiologic Consequences

Hypoxemia, hypercapnia, acidemia, which are confirmed by arterial blood gases.

Clinical Findings

Tachypnea, tachycardia, hypertension or hypotension, cyanosis, confusion, coma, papilledema, asterixis, cardiac arrhythmias, and headaches.

Pulmonary function tests show decreased VC, peak inspiratory flow.

Arterial blood gas determination and examination of the patient are the best ways of determining ventilatory failure.

Treatment

Oxygen therapy, ventilatory support, correction of acid—base balance, and treatment of the underlying cause.

Caution must be taken when oxygen therapy is given to COPD patients.

Ventilatory Failure in Chronic Obstructive Pulmonary Disease (COPD)

Meaning

Patients with COPD have already compromised physical and clinical features, which can hide acute ventilatory failure, up to the point of being life-threatening. Deterioration of clinical findings should alert you to impending problems.

Possible Causes

Depressed central drive caused by drugs (sedatives), excessive use of oxygen, or metabolic alkalosis. Other possible causes include acute bronchitis, pneumonia, allergies, and dehydration.

150 □ Respiratory Facts

Clinical Findings

Decreased flow rates (pulmonary function tests), positive for overuse of sedatives, changes in sputum production, chest x-rays positive for pneumonia, positive for Gram's stain, and possible cardiovascular effects.

Treatment

Therapy should be directed for rehydration. Reduce or stop sedatives. Control oxygen percentage. Provide chest physical therapy, nebulizer or IPPB therapy, and nutritional support.

BIBLIOGRAPHY

The works listed below are also suggested readings that will give the reader more information concerning the chapter content.

Abels, LF: Mosby's Manual of Critical Care. CV Mosby, St. Louis, 1979.

Byrne, CJ: Laboratory Tests. Addison-Wesley, Menlo Park, CA, 1986.

Daily, EK: Techniques in Bedside Hemodynamic Monitoring, ed 3. CV Mosby, St. Louis, 1985.

Gylys, B and Wedding, MH: Medical Terminology: A Systems Approach, ed 2. FA Davis, Philadelphia, 1988.

Des Jardins, T: Clinical Manifestations of Respiratory Diseases. Year Book Medical Publishers, Chicago, 1984.

Kacmarck, RM: The Essentials of Respiratory Therapy, ed 2. Year Book Medical Publishers, Chicago, 1985.

Lough, WT, Rawson, JE: Newborn Respiratory Care. Year Book Medical Publishers, Chicago, 1979.

McPherson, SP: Respiratory Therapy Equipment, ed 3. CV Mosby, St. Louis, 1985.

Moser, KM: Respiratory Emergencies. CV Mosby, St. Louis, 1982.

Patterson, R: Current Drug Handbook. WB Saunders, Philadelphia, 1986.

Roberts, JT: Fundamentals of Tracheal Intubation. Grune & Stratton, New York, 1983.

Wilkins, WL: Clinical Assessment in Respiratory Care. CV Mosby, St. Louis, 1985.

NOTES

5 **Airways and Ventilators**

Types of Blades Used for Intubation

MacIntosh

Miller

Specialized Blades

Curved

Bizzarri-Guiffrida

Siker

Fink

Straight

Guedel

Whitehead

Bennett

Tube Size

Indications for Mechanical Ventilation

Settings on Mechanical Ventilators

Modes

Control

Assist/Control

Intermittent Mandatory Ventilation (IMV)

Synchronized Intermittent Mandatory
Ventilation (SIMV)

Tidal Volume and Ventilatory Rate Settings

Monitoring the Ventilator

Ventilator Math

Ventilator Discontinuance and Weaning

Criteria for Discontinuance

Troubleshooting Mechanical Ventilators

High Pressure

Possible Causes

Possible Corrections

Low Pressure

Possible Causes

Possible Corrections

Oxygen Fail

Possible Causes

Possible Corrections

ARTIFICIAL AIRWAYS

There are four main indications for an artificial airway:
1. To prevent or relieve airway obstruction
2. To protect the airway from aspiration or collapse
3. To facilitate suctioning
4. To provide a sealed system for mechanical ventilation
There are nine types of airways:
1. Oropharyngeal
2. Nasopharyngeal
3. Esophageal
4. Oral endotracheal tube
5. Nasal endotracheal tube
6. Tracheostomy tube
7. Fenestrated tracheostomy tube
8. Talking tracheostomy tube
9. Tracheal button

Oropharyngeal (Fig. 5–1)

Sometimes called *S* or *J tube*. Relieves obstruction caused by the tongue. It is adequate for comatose patients only. Helps in suctioning. Good oral hygiene is necessary with any kind of airway and should be performed every 4 hours with careful inspection of the mouth for signs of pressure spots. Care should be taken with patients who are awake for possible aspiration due to gag reflex. This tube is not to be used for mechanical ventilation support.

Nasopharyngeal

Prevents or relieves obstruction caused by tongue or soft tissue. Extends from the nose to the hypopharnyx. It is adequate for comatose or alert patients. Aids in suctioning. Humidification is required. Tube should be rotated every 48 hours. The use of a water-soluble lubricant will aid in the insertion. This tube is not to be used for mechanical ventilation support.

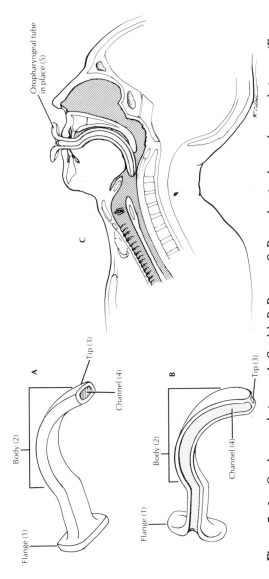

Figure 5–1. Oropharyngeal airways. A, Guedel. B, Berman. C, Proper location for oropharyngeal airways. (From Eubanks, DH and Bone, RC: Comprehensive Respiratory Care: A Learning System. CV Mosby, St. Louis, 1985, p 491, with permission.)

Flange (1)

Body (2)

Tip (3)

Channel (4)

A

Flange (1)

Body (2)

Channel (4)

Tip (3)

B

Oropharyngeal tube in place (5)

C

Esophageal Obturator (Fig. 5 – 2)

Not to be used with mechanical ventilation. To be used only in case of an emergency in unconscious patients. Prevents aspiration of gastric contents. Not to be used on children. Hazards include inadvertent endotracheal intubation and esophageal trauma. You should intubate before removing the obturator.

Oral Endotracheal Tube (Fig. 5 – 3)

This is the airway of choice in an *emergency*. Can be accomplished faster than nasotracheal intubation because of direct visualization of the chords. Sometimes poorly tolerated by patients who are awake. The patient can bite into the tube and occlude the airway. Inadvertent extubation sometimes happens. Sometimes the tube can be hard to stabilize. The length of time an oral tube should be left in place is *debatable* — anywhere from 2 days to 6 weeks. If the first attempt at

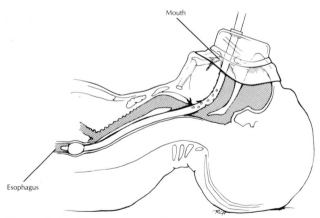

Figure 5–2. Proper placement for an esophageal obturator. (From Eubanks, DH and Bone, RC: Comprehensive Respiratory Care: A Learning System. CV Mosby, St. Louis, 1985, p 493, with permission.)

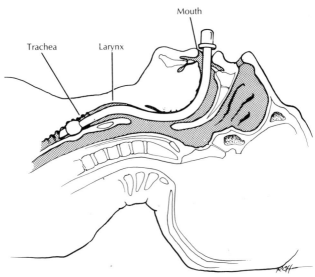

Figure 5-3. Proper placement for an oral endotracheal tube. (From Eubanks, DH and Bone, RC: Comprehensive Respiratory Care: A Learning System. CV Mosby, St. Louis, 1985, p 493, with permission.)

intubation is unsuccessful, other attempts can be made only after reoxygenation of the patient.

Nasotracheal Tube (Fig. 5-4)

This tube is better tolerated by the patient. It is easier to stabilize. A major problem is nasal mucosal necrosis. The use of a water-soluble lubricant makes passing the tube easier and with less trauma to the patient.

Tracheostomy Tube

There are three main indications for use of a tracheostomy tube: when long-term respiratory support is needed, when oral

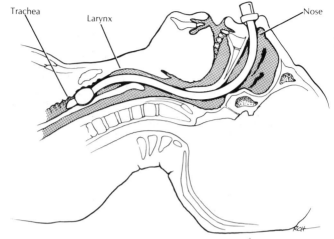

Figure 5–4. Proper placement for a nasotracheal tube. (From Eubanks, DH and Bone, RC: Comprehensive Respiratory Care: A Learning System. CV Mosby, St. Louis, 1985, p 493, with permission.)

and nasal intubation is no longer tolerated due to possible necrosis, and to bypass an obstruction of the upper airway. Tracheostomy tubes are the best tolerated of all airways. They can be cuffed or uncuffed. Uncuffed tubes should be avoided in the hospitalized patient because of difficulty in resuscitation if needed.

Fenestrated Tracheostomy Tubes

This type of tube has an opening in the outer cannula, but when the inner cannula is in place it acts as a regular tracheostomy tube. The fenestrated tube aids in the weaning process by allowing air to pass through the upper airway, which allows phonation.

Polyvinylchloride (PVC) Tubes

Most commonly used material in endotracheal tubes; cannot be gas cleaned; are mostly for one-time use.

Silicone Rubber (Silastic) Tubes

Low tissue toxicity; opaque; very flexible.

Airway Cuffs

The best type of cuff is the high residual volume or low-pressure cuffs, cylindrical shape, large diameter, with residual volumes of 12 to 15 ml. The cuff inflates evenly owing to large contact area.

High-pressure airway cuffs have a small contact area with the trachea, providing high cuff-to-wall pressure; exceed safe limits due to low residual volume; may cause significant tracheal damage even when used for short periods of time.

INTUBATION

General Provisions

General provisions include proper position (surgical beds or beds with removable headboards are desired); often the shoulders must be raised slightly with a pillow or roll. Light (good room lighting is necessary to observe retractions, cyanosis, and foreign matter in the mouth). Suction is of the utmost importance and must be immediately at hand. There should be a number of suction catheters and a tonsil suction at the bedside. A mask, bag, and oxygen should be on hand at all times. In most cases airway insertion is not a one-person job. Persons assisting with intubations or any type of airway care should be familiar with all equipment and understand their use.

Checklist of Instruments

The following is a checklist of instruments:

Bite blocks, sizes small, medium, and large
Tongue depressors, two or more
Oral airways, sizes 0 – 4
Nasal airways, sizes small, medium, and large
Laryngoscope (check batteries)
Laryngoscope blades, both straight and curved (check lightbulbs)
Magill forceps for nasal intubation
Tubes, a good supply with a wide selection of sizes
Stylet to be used as a guide (Care should be taken that the end of the stylet does not go beyond the end of the tube.)
Syringe, 10 – 20 ml, to be used to inflate the cuff
Hemostat (For old-type tube that does not have a self-sealing cuff, the hemostat should have a covering to prevent cutting of the pilot tube.)
Suction catheters, a large supply at hand
Tape, for taping tubes
Benzoin, helps the tape stay on the skin

SUCTIONING

The most important thing to do when suctioning is to preoxygenate and postoxygenate.

Indications

Indications for suctioning include airway obstruction (rales, rhonchi, and wheezes), as an aid to help the patient cough, and for bronchial hygiene.

Hazards

Hazards when suctioning include tachycardia, bradycardia, hypoxia, infection, arrhythmia, and trauma.

The mouth and nose are considered contaminated and you should not pass a catheter from the mouth or nose to the endotracheal tube.

Checklist of Instruments
Suction catheters of appropriate size
Sterile disposable gloves
Oxygen source, flow meter, and tubing
Hand resuscitator
Vacuum source and tubing

TYPES OF BLADES USED
FOR INTUBATION

MacIntosh. A curved blade, size 87 mm to 158 mm
(Figs. 5–5, 5–6).
Miller. A straight blade, size 75 mm to 205 mm (See
Figs. 5–5, 5–6).

Specialized Blades

Curved

Bizzarri-Guiffrida. The left ridge is removed for use
on patients with limited mouth opening, short thick neck, or
when the larynx is in an extreme anterior position (Fig. 5–7).
Siker. Has a stainless-steel surface that acts as a mirror.
The surface does invert the image, making the blade difficult to
use. The blade is used on routine patients (Fig. 5–8).
Fink. Is reduced in size at the hook end. The curvature
at the tip is increased.

Straight

Guedel. Has a 72-degree angle between the blade and
the handle.
Whitehead. Reduced left-sided ridge, reducing pressure against the upper teeth.
Bennett. Reduced left-sided ridge plus it has a 72-de-
gree angle between the blade and the handle.

TUBE SIZE

Tables 5–1 through 5–4 discuss tube size.

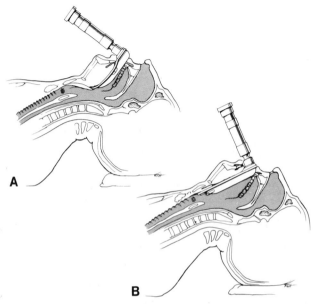

Figure 5 – 5. Proper placement of a curved (MacIntosh) blade (*A*), and of a straight (Miller) blade (*B*). (From Eubanks, DH and Bone, RC: Comprehensive Respiratory Care: A Learning System. CV Mosby, St. Louis, 1985, p 509, with permission.)

INDICATIONS FOR MECHANICAL VENTILATION

There are three main reasons for placing a patient on mechanical ventilation: apnea, acute ventilatory failure, and impending ventilatory failure. Placing a patient on mechanical ventilation should not be taken lightly. Patient assessment and proper lab value assessment can be a great aid in determining if a patient is to be placed on a ventilator. Table 5 – 5 provides a list of clinical measurement normals and measurements when you may need to institute mechanical ventilation.

SETTINGS ON MECHANICAL VENTILATORS

Modes

Control

Patient is totally dependent on the ventilator for rate and tidal volume. The patient is unable to control any aspect of ventilation.

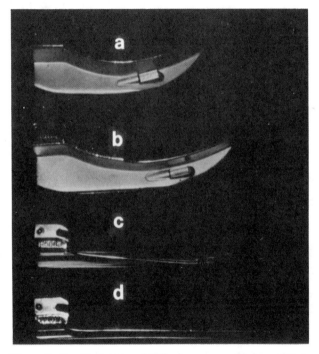

Figure 5–6. MacIntosh and Miller laryngoscope blades. *a*, MacIntosh No. 3 (usual adult size); *b*, MacIntosh No. 4; *c*, Miller No. 2 (usual adult size); *d*, Miller No. 3. (From Roberts, JJ: Fundamentals of Tracheal Intubation. Grune & Stratton, New York, 1983, p. 50, with permission.)

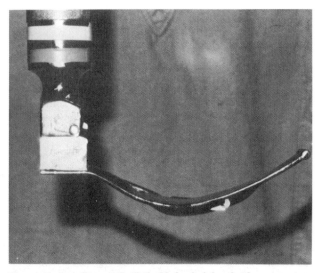

Figure 5–7. Bizzarri-Guiffrida blade. Left-hand ridge present on MacIntosh blade has been removed. (From Roberts, JJ: Fundamentals of Tracheal Intubation. Grune & Stratton, New York, 1983, p 51, with permission.)

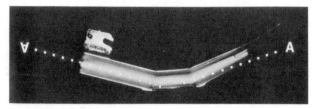

Figure 5–8. Siker blade. Mirrored surface reflects inverted image from anterior larynx. You must practice using this blade during normal laryngoscopy; do not expect to learn on a difficult intubation. (From Roberts, JJ: Fundamentals of Tracheal Intubation. Grune & Stratton, New York, 1983, with permission.)

Table 5-1. ESTIMATED ENDOTRACHEAL TUBE SIZE
AND
SUCTION CATHETERS

Patient's age	Suction Catheter (French)	Endotracheal Tube (Internal Diameter — mm)
Newborn	5-6	3.0
6 months	6	3.5
18 months	8	4.0
3 years	8	4.5
5 years	8	5.0
6 years	8	5.5
8 years	10	6.0
12 years	10	6.5
16 years	10	7.0
Adult female	12	8.0-8.5
Adult male	14	8.5-9.0

Assist/Control

Tidal volume is controlled by the ventilator with the control mode set at a back-up rate. If the patient fails to trigger an assist breath, the patient will receive a control breath. It should be noted that the patient will receive the same tidal volume regardless of how the breath is given.

Intermittent Mandatory Ventilation (IMV)

Combines controlled ventilation while allowing the patient to breathe spontaneously at his own rate and tidal volume between controlled breaths.

Synchronized Intermittent Mandatory Ventilation (SIMV)

Combines assist/control ventilation with spontaneous breathing. This is about the same as IMV but helps in preventing mechanical ventilated breaths being given at the same time

Table 5–2. DIMENSIONS OF LOW-
PRESSURE CUFFED ADULT
TRACHEOSTOMY TUBES

Size	Inner Diameter	Outer Diameter	Length
Kamen-Wilkinson (Bivona)			
5	6.0	8.7	70
6	7.0	10.0	84
7	8.0	11.0	90
8	9.0	12.3	105
9	9.5	13.3	105
Lanz			
5	6.0	8.0	73
6	7.0	9.0	78
7	8.0	11.0	84
8	9.0	12.0	88
9	10.0	13.0	92
Portex			
6	7.5	10	76
7	8.2	11	83
8	9.0	12	91
9	9.7	13	96
Shiley			
4	5.0	8.5	60
6	7.0	10.0	68
8	8.5	12.0	71
10	9.0	13.0	71

as a spontaneous breath taken by the patient. Also called *stacking*.

Tidal Volume and Ventilatory Rate Settings

Large tidal volumes and low rates will increase alveolar ventilation, improve distribution of ventilation, and decrease

Table 5–3. TRACHEOSTOMY TUBE AND CUFF SIZE CONVERSION CHART

Jackson	Outer Diameter	French	Inner Diameter
00	4.3	13	2.5
0	5.0	15	3.0
1	5.5	16.5	3.5
2	6.0	18	4.0
3	7.0	21	4.5–5.0
4	8.0	24	5.5
5	9.0	27	6.0–6.5
6	10.0	30	7.0
7	11.0	33	7.5–8.0
8	12.0	36	8.5
9	13.0	39	9.0–9.5
10	14.0	42	10.0
11	15.0	45	10.5–11.0
12	16.0	48	11.5

mean intrathoracic pressure. Tidal volume settings range from 8 to 15 ml/kg, while respiratory rates run from 4 to 12 breaths/minute (for an adult). Note that patients with chronic restrictive pulmonary disease use tidal volumes in the 5 to 10 ml/kg range and respiratory rates of 20 to 38/minute.

The patient's response to mechanical ventilation should be checked at the same time as the ventilator. Emotional and mental status of the patient should never be overlooked.

MONITORING THE VENTILATOR

Once the patient is on the ventilator, monitoring of the patient should be done every 2 hours or when a malfunction is suspected. When checking a ventilator, care should be given not to overlook any control, tubing, or the patient. *A check-off list of things to monitor follows:*
Tidal volume delivered, set, exhaled, and spontaneous
Respiratory rate, set rate, and spontaneous rate
FI_{O_2} ordered and delivered

Table 5-4. APPROXIMATE EQUIVALENT OF
ENDOTRACHEAL
TUBE SIZING METHODS

Internal	External	Magill	French	Equivalent (Cuff)
2.5	4.0		12	
3.0	4.5	00	12-14	
3.5	5.0	00	14-16	$3/16''$
4.0	5.5	0-1	16-18	$3/16''$
4.5	6.0	1-2	18-20	$3/16''$
5.0	6.5	1-2	20-22	$3/16''$ or $1/4''$
5.5	7.0	3-4	22	$1/4''$
6.0	8.0	3-4	24	$1/4''$
6.5	8.5	4-5	26	$1/4''$
7.0	9.0	5-6	28	$5/16''$
7.5	9.5	6-7	30	$5/16''$
8.0	10.0	7-8	32	$5/16''$
8.5	11.5	8	34	$3/8''$
9.0	12.0	9-10	36	$3/8''$
9.5	12.5	9-10	38	$3/8''$
10.0	13.0	10-11	40	$7/16''$
10.5	13.5	10-11	42	$7/16''$
11.0	14.5	11-12	42-44	$1/2''$
11.5	15.0	11-12	44-46	$1/2''$

Mode of ventilation, control, assist/control, IMV, and SIMV
Maximum inspiratory pressure, plateau pressure, and PEEP
levels
Inspiratory flow rate
Temperature of inspired air
Humidifier water level
Alarm settings for apnea, pressure, volume, rate, oxygen, etc.
Patient comfort
Proper endotracheal tube position and cuff inflation pressure
Empty water-filled tubing
Vital signs
ECGs

Table 5-5. CLINICAL MEASUREMENT NORMALS AND MEASUREMENTS INDICATING NEED FOR VENTILATION

Clinical Measurement	Normal	May Need to Institute Ventilation
Blood Gas Tensions		
pH	7.34 – 7.45	<7.25
Pa_{CO_2}	34 – 45	>55 with pH <7.25
Pa_{O_2}	80 – 100 (on .21%)	<50 and pH <7.25
Pulmonary Function Studies		
Tidal volume (ml/kg)	5 – 8	<5
Vital capacity (ml/kg)	65 – 75	<10 or 2 × Vt
Forced expiratory volume in 1 second (ml/kg)	50 – 60	<10
Respiratory rate	12 – 20	>40 or absent
Negative inspiratory force	>20 – 30	<20
Physiologic Oxygenation Studies		
$[P_{(A-a)O_2}]$ breathing 100%	25 – 65	>350
$(Pa_{O_2}/P_{A_{O_2}})$ ratio	0.75	<0.15
$(Qs/Qt)\%$	<5%	20% – 30%
$(Vd/Vt)\%$	.25% – .45%	>.50%

173

Monitoring the patient and ventilator will help detect problems earlier when they are easier to correct. Do not get in the habit of just doing a "quickie" ventilator check.

Remember the goals of mechanical ventilation:
1. To decrease the work of breathing
2. To improve $\dot{V}/\dot{Q}$ ratio
3. To improve V_A
4. To improve distribution of ventilation

VENTILATOR MATH

To find I : E time when you know Vt, peak flow, and rate:

$$60 \text{ sec} \sqrt{\dfrac{\text{L/sec}}{\text{Peak flow L/minute}}}$$

$$\text{L/sec} \sqrt{\dfrac{\text{Inspiratory time needed to deliver set tidal volume}}{\text{Tidal volume in liters}}}$$

$$\text{Rate} \sqrt{\dfrac{\text{Total cycle time}}{60 \text{ sec}}}$$

$$\dfrac{\text{Total cycle time}}{- \text{ Inspiratory time}}$$
$$\text{Expiratory time}$$

Example:
Given Vt .600 L, peak flow 30 L/minute, and rate 10/minute:

$$60 \sqrt{\dfrac{.5}{30.0}}$$

$$.5 \sqrt{\dfrac{1.2}{.600}}$$

$$10 \sqrt{\dfrac{6}{60}}$$

$$\dfrac{6.0 \text{ Total cycle time}}{- 1.2 \text{ Inspiratory time}}$$
$$4.8 \text{ Expiratory time}$$

Another way to find I : E time if you know I : E ratio and rate without knowing peak flow:

$$\text{Rate} \overline{\smash{\big)}\,\underset{\text{60 sec}}{\overset{\text{6 sec total cycle time}}{}}}$$

$$\text{I} + \text{E ratio}$$

$$\text{Total of I} + \text{E ratio} \overline{\smash{\big)}\,\underset{\text{Total cycle time}}{\overset{\text{Inspiratory time}}{}}}$$

$$\begin{array}{r} \text{Total cycle time} \\ - \ \text{Inspiratory time} \\ \hline \text{Expiratory time} \end{array}$$

Example:

Given an I : E ratio of 1 : 2 and rate 10:

$$10 \overline{\smash{\big)}\,\underset{60}{\overset{\text{6 sec total cycle time}}{}}}$$

$$1 + 2 = 3$$

$$3 \overline{\smash{\big)}\,\underset{\text{6 total cycle time}}{\overset{\text{2 sec inspiratory time}}{}}}$$

$$\begin{array}{r} \text{6 sec total cycle time} \\ - \ \text{2 sec inspiratory time} \\ \hline \text{4 sec expiratory time} \end{array}$$

To find exhaled minute volume:

$$\text{Vt} \times \text{rate} = \dot{V}_E$$

To find peak flow rate:

$$\dot{V}_E \times (\text{I} + \text{E ratio}) = \text{MPF}$$

To find resistance:

$$\text{Resistance} = \frac{\text{Maximum inspiratory pressure} - \text{Plateau pressure}}{\text{Flow rate}}$$

To find patient's tidal volume:

Patient's weight in kg $\times$ 8 – 15 ml/kg = Vt

(8 – 15 ml/kg is only an estimation.)

To correct Pa_{CO_2}:

$$\dot{V}_E = \frac{\text{Present } \dot{V}_E \times \text{present } Pa_{CO_2}}{\text{Desired } Pa_{CO_2}}$$

or

$$\text{New rate} = \frac{\text{Present rate} \times \text{present } Pa_{CO_2}}{\text{Desired } Pa_{CO_2}}$$

VENTILATOR DISCONTINUANCE AND WEANING

Criteria for Discontinuance

Reversal of the pathophysiologic condition

No active acute pulmonary disease process

Stable vital signs

Optimal nutritional status (for long-term ventilator patients)

No arrhythmias, or if present can be managed

Normal renal function with proper electrolyte and fluid balance

Adequate gas exchange

Intrapulmonary shunt of <20% – 25%

Adequate bedside pulmonary function tests: VC > or equal to 10 – 15 ml/kg; Vt spontaneous 3 – 5 ml/kg; NIF > – 20 to 25 cmH$_2$O

There are many other techniques for weaning a patient. Use the NOTES page to write in your own method.

TROUBLESHOOTING MECHANICAL VENTILATORS

Following is a list of ventilator problems, patient problems, and possible causes, and therapist decisions for corrections of these problems.

High Pressure

Possible Causes

These include airway obstruction, patient circuit collapse or kinked tubing, coughing, possible tension pneumothorax, improper alarm setting, high resistance, decreased lung compliance, and/or the patient "fighting" the ventilator.

Possible Corrections

Suction the patient, unkink tube and clear any obstruction from tubing, give bronchodilator therapy, check breath sounds and x-ray looking for pneumothorax and possible pneumonia, check arterial blood gases for hypoxia, reassure the patient, and look for stomach distention that would put pressure on the diaphragm, resulting in an increase in airway pressure.

Low Pressure

Possible Causes

These include leak or unattached tubing, leak around humidifier, leak around the patient's endotracheal tube, poor cuff inflation, peak flows that are too low, and incorrect tidal volumes (too low).

Possible Corrections

Reconnect tubing, tighten humidifier, change or reposition endotracheal tube, correct cuff pressures, adjust peak flow to meet or exceed patient demand, and correct for the patient's tidal volume.

Oxygen Fail

Possible Causes

These include oxygen not connected to ventilator, dirty oxygen intake filter, and improper oxygen alarm setting.

Possible Corrections

Reconnect or connect oxygen line to a 50 psi source, clean or replace oxygen filter, and correct alarm setting.

Ratio

Possible Causes

These include inspiratory time longer than expiratory time, peak flow setting too low while rate too high, and the use of an inspiratory phase that is too long with a fast rate.

Possible Corrections

Change inspiratory time or adjust peak flow, check inspiratory phase, or hold.

Failure to Cycle

Possible Causes

These include low inspiratory demand during assist/control mode, ventilator malfunction (circuit breaker tripped), and possible power failure or disconnect.

Possible Corrections

Adjust sensitivity setting, reset circuit breaker, and reconnect power source or hand ventilate patient until power is restored.

Temperature

Possible Causes

These include overheating due to too low or no gas flow, sensor malfunction, sensor picking up outside air flow (from heaters, open doors or windows, air conditioners), and improper water levels.

Possible Corrections

Check gas flow, test or replace sensor, protect sensor from outside sources that would interfere with readings, and check water levels.

VENTILATORS

Emerson 3-PV Post-Op

Electrically powered, time or patient cycled, rotary-driven piston, single-circuit ventilator that was designed to be volume limited.

Specifications

Tidal volume, 0 to 2000 ml
Inspiratory time, 0.4 to 3.0 sec
Expiratory time, 0.4 to 3.0 sec
Approximate rate, 10 to 50 breaths/minute
Assist effort, -1 cmH$_2$O
Pressure limit, 40 to 140 cmH$_2$O
Sighs, adjustable
Alarms, there are no alarms systems

Emerson IMV

Electrically powered, rotary-driven piston, single-circuit ventilator designed to be volume limited.

Specifications

Tidal volume, 0 to 2000 ml
Total cycle time, 2.3 to 5.0 sec
Approximate rate, 1 breath/5 minutes to 26 breaths
Pressure limit, 40 to 120 cmH$_2$O
Alarms, there are no standard alarm systems
The Emerson ventilator can be set up with a number of alarm systems. Emerson parts can be obtained at most hardware stores.

Engstrom

Electrically powered, rotary-driven piston, double-circuit, time-cycled, time- and volume-limited controllers.

Specifications

Minute volume, 0 to 50 L/minute
Rate, 12 to 35 (300 series) or 10 to 30 (150–200 series)
I : E ratio, fixed at 1 : 2
Pressure limit, 30, 60, and 90 cmH$_2$O (300 series) to 35 to 70 cmH$_2$O (150–200 series)
Alarms, disconnect and low pressure

Bennett MA-1

Electrically powered, low-pressure driven, double-circuit, compressor-powered bellows, volume limited, patient or time cycled.

Specifications

Tidal volume, 0 to 2200 ml (normal and sigh)
Rate, 6 to 60 or <1 to 60 for IMV
Peak flow, 15 to 100 L/minute
Pressure limit, 20 to 80 cmH$_2$O
Alarms, I : E ratio, high pressure, oxygen (low volume can be added)

A number of alarm systems have been added to the Bennett MA-1. Spirometers for exhaled volumes and Bunn alarms are the more common systems.

Bennett MA-2

Electrically powered and controlled, low-pressure driven, double-circuit, compressor-powered bellows, designed to be volume limited.

Specifications

Modes, CMV and IMV
Tidal volume, 0 to 2200 ml
CMV rate, 3 to 60 breaths/minute
IMV rate, 1 breath for 3 minutes to 30 minutes
Peak flow, 15 to 125 L/minute
PEEP/CPAP, 0 to 45 cmH_2O
Pressure limit, 20 to 120 cmH_2O
Alarms, oxygen, high and low pressure, I:E ratio alarm

Bennett MA 2+2

Electrically powered and controlled, low-pressure driven, double-circuit, compressor-powered bellows, volume limited.

Specifications

Essentially the same as the Bennett MA-2, with only 3 design improvements:
1. Adjustable low inspiratory pressure alarm from 2 to 80 cmH_2O
2. Automatic bellows reset following patient disconnection
3. Universal humidifier mount

Ohio CCV-2 SIMV

Electrically powered and controlled, low-pressure driven, rotary blower, double circuit with bellows, designed to be volume limited, patient or time cycled on.

Specifications

Tidal volume, 200 to 2000 ml
Flow rate, above 200 L/minute
Expiratory time, 1 to 10 sec
Rate, 5 to 40 breaths/minute; 4 to 120 sec expiratory time for
  IMV, SIMV
Pressure limit, 30 to 100 cmH_2O

PEEP, up to 40 cmH_2O
Alarms, low pressure, high pressure, fail to cycle, loss of power,
    oxygen

Siemens 900B

Pneumatically powered, electronically controlled, spring-
driven bellows, designed to be time limited and minute volume
preset, patient or time cycled.

Specifications

Minute volume, 0.5 to > 25 L/minute
Rate, 6 to 60/minute on assist-control (a/c) or 6 to 60 divided
    by 2, 5, or 10 on IMV
Pressure limit, 100 cmH_2O, same as machine
Alarms, high and low minimum volume, press limit, power
    failure

Siemens 900c

Pneumatically powered, electronically controlled, low-
pressure drive, single-circuit, spring-driven bellows, patient,
time, volume, or pressure cycled with pressure support.

Specifications

Minute volume, 0.5 to 40 L/minute
Rate, 5 to 120 (SIMV .5 to 40 L/minute)
PEEP, 0 to 50 cmH_2O
Pressure limit, 16 to 120 cmH_2O
Alarms, oxygen %, gas supply, power fail, minute volume, press
    limit, apnea

Air Shield Oracle Volume Ventilator

Microprocessor and electronically controlled, pneumatically powered, volume-limited, minute-volume ventilator.

Specifications

Rate, 1 to 60 breaths/minute
Tidal volume, 200 to 2500 ml
PEEP, 0 to 32 cmH_2O
Pressure limited, 10 to 120 cmH_2O
Minute volume, 0.2 to 35 L/minute
Peak flow, 10 to 120 L/minute
Alarms, high pressure, low pressure, patient disconnect, apnea, low minimum volume, high rate

Bear I and II

Pneumatically and electrically powered, electrically controlled ventilator that is volume limited, time or patient cycled, time or pressure limited.

Bear I Specifications

Tidal volume, 100 to 2000 ml
Rate, 5 to 60 or 0.5 to 6/minute with divided by 10 switch
Pressure limit, 0 to 100 cmH_2O
Peak flow, 20 to 120 L/minute
PEEP, 0 to 30 cmH_2O
Alarms, low presssure and exhaled volume, PEEP/CPAP, apnea, ventilator inoperative

Bear II Specifications

Tidal volume, 100 to 2000 ml
Rate, 0.5 to 60 breaths/minute
Pressure limit, 0 to 120 cmH_2O
Peak flow, 10 to 120 L/minute
PEEP, 0 to 50 cmH_2O
Alarms, low pressure (inspiratory), low exhaled volume, low PEEP/CPAP, apnea, ventilator inoperative
The internal compressor is automatically turned on if source of gas pressure is inadequate or absent.

Puritan Bennett 7200 Microprocessor

Electrically powered, high-pressure drive, single-circuit, electronically controlled, proportional solenoid-driven ventilator that is volume limited, patient or time cycled.

Specifications

Tidal volume, 0.10 to 2.50 L
Rate, 0.5 to 70 breaths/minute
High pressure limit, 10 to 120 cmH$_2$O
Alarms, I : E ratio, high rate, low inspiratory pressure, apnea, low PEEP/CPAP, high pressure, low volume, low exhaled minimum volume, low gas pressure

Bio Med IC-5

Electronically controlled, high-pressure drive, single-circuit, solenoid- and restrictor-module-powered ventilator designed to be volume limited.

Specifications

Tidal volume, 50 to 3000 ml
Flow, 5 to 120 L/minute
Rate, 5 to 150 breaths/minute
SIMV rate, 0.5 to 30 breaths/minute
PEEP/CPAP, 0 to 35 cmH$_2$O
Alarms, fail to cycle, low gas supply, low battery, peak pressure, O$_2$%, exhaled minimum volume
See Chapter 6 for home care ventilators and related information.
See Chapter 7 for infant ventilators and related information.

BIBLIOGRAPHY

The works listed below are also suggested readings that will give the reader more information concerning the chapter content.

Burton, GG: Respiratory Care: A Guide to Respiratory Therapy. JB Lippincott, Philadelphia, 1984.

Kacmarck, RM: The Essentials of Respiratory Therapy, ed 2. Year Book Medical Publishers, Chicago, 1985.

McPherson, SP: Respiratory Therapy Equipment, ed 3. CV Mosby, St. Louis, 1985.

Roberts, JT: Fundamentals of Tracheal Intubation. Grune & Stratton, New York, 1983.

Shoup, CA: Laboratory Exercises in Respiratory Therapy, ed 2. CV Mosby, St. Louis, 1983.

NOTES

6

Respiratory Home Care

DEFINITION OF RESPIRATORY HOME CARE

In 1943, Dr. Albert Andrews Jr. talked about home care. "Oxygen therapy in the home is feasible and its use is steadily increasing. The therapy can be just as efficient in the home as in the hospital. . . ." With the prospective payment system started in 1983, home care has again become a large and growing business, with hospitals and even department stores getting involved.

GOALS FOR HOME CARE OXYGEN THERAPY

To use low-flow oxygen, keeping Pa_{O_2} near 55 to 60 mmHg, to try to relieve dyspnea while at rest, to reduce pulmonary hypertension, and to maintain other nonpulmonary organs in a state of relative homeostasis.

OXYGEN SYSTEMS USED IN HOME CARE

There are three main oxygen systems used in home care: oxygen cylinders, liquid oxygen, and oxygen concentrators.

Oxygen Cylinders

These can provide high flow rates, need little maintenance, have 100% concentrations, are ready for immediate use, and do not need electrical outlets for operation.

Some of their limitations are constant refills, large storage area, heavy tanks, limited patient mobility, and hazards due to high-pressure contents.

Liquid Oxygen*

These systems have two types of reservoirs. The main unit can hold 18, 28, or 40 liters of liquid oxygen; the second, a portable unit, can hold 1, 2, or 3 liters of liquid oxygen. Both units require very little maintenance. The portable unit can be refilled from the main unit and is lightweight.

Limitations include problems of refilling a cold liquid gas, expense of refills, evaporation of liquid gas even when not in use, and time limits of both units before refills are required.

Oxygen Concentrators

These are the least expensive if used over 18 hours a day. No refilling is needed and there is very little maintenance. Smaller units are portable, and most look like home furniture.

Limitations include possible power failure, required back-up systems, and low flows (the higher the flow, the lower the

---

*New liquid systems are 21, 31, and 41 liters.

oxygen percentage); oxygen percentages will vary with liter flow and make of the unit.

HOME CARE VENTILATORS

In the past few years, the number of patients going home still needing respiratory care has increased. A few of these patients need ventilator care. The use of home ventilator care has been debated over the past few years, based on the fact that mechanical ventilators require high technological skills and that a patient's family does not have the skills required to provide the care needed. Manufacturers of ventilators for use in the home understand this problem and have tried to simplify the ventilators so that the patient's family can obtain the skill necessary to operate the ventilator safely.

There are a number of home care ventilators on the market at this time. The operational characteristics, safeguards, and accessories of some home care ventilators now on the market follow.

Thompson (Puritan Bennett) MV Maxivent

Maxivent is an electrically powered ventilator, designed for negative-pressure application.

Operational Characteristics

Controls — negative-pressure and positive-pressure mode; this control activates pressures from -70 to $+80$ cmH$_2$O.
Rate — 8 to 24 breaths/minute
Power — on/off toggle switch
Alarm — delay good for 1 minute

Patient/Operator Safeguards

Alarms. On/off (ventilator) *alarm* — green light indicates power is being supplied to ventilator. *Low-pressure audible alarm* — if pressure drops below -10 cmH$_2$O in the negative mode or below $+10$ cmH$_2$O in the positive mode for longer than 12 seconds the alarm will sound. *Fail to cycle alarm* — an audible alarm that will sound if the ventilator fails to cycle within 12 seconds. *Power failure* — an audible alarm activated by an internal battery within 12 seconds after loss of AC power. The manometer is an integral pressure gauge calibrated in cmH$_2$O from -80 to $+80$ cmH$_2$O.

Power Source.   120 AC, 60 Hz, 2.4 amps, 160 watts.

Optional Accessories

Pneumobelt, chest sheet, patient call switch, cascade humidifier, and body wrap.

Thompson (Puritan Bennett) M3000XA

A highly sophisticated portable ventilator that can be powered by 120 AC or 12 DC. In the event of an external power failure in the AC mode, the ventilator will automatically switch to an internal battery, which can support the ventilator for up to 3 hours without recharging. This unit provides assist/control, control, or IMV modes of ventilation. Adjustable sighs provide 3 to 4 breaths at a rate of approximately 6 sigh breaths/hour. Oxygen accumulator is available for attachment to deliver up to 100% oxygen.

Operational Characteristics

Control mode ventilator delivers breaths at preselected intervals at preselected volumes, unless the pressure limit has been reached.

Assist mode ventilator cycles in response to the patient's inspiratory effort and delivers the preselected volume, unless the adjustable pressure limit has been reached.

IMV mode has an operator-adjustable IMV rate as low as 2.5 breaths/minute.

Controls

Normal volume rotary control is adjustable from 200 to 3000 ml.

Normal pressure limit rotary control permits adjustments of maximum pressure limit from +15 to +65 cmH_2O.

Breaths per minute rotary control is adjustable up to 30 breaths/minute.

Inspiratory time rotary control adjusts inspiratory time from 1.0 to 3.0 seconds.

Sigh volume rotary control adjusts sigh volumes from 200 to 3000 ml.

Sigh pressure limit rotary control is adjustable from 15 to 65 cmH_2O.

Sigh has a 3-position toggle switch for pressure-limited sigh, volume-limited sigh, or sigh off.

Manual sigh is a red push button that will activate a sigh breath.

BPM inspiration toggle switch dedicates analog display to breaths per minute or inspiratory time in seconds.

IMV/CON/assist is a 3-position toggle switch that dedicates ventilator to one of the three modes of operation.

Low-pressure rotary control adjusts low-pressure alarm limits from +10 to +35 cmH_2O

Time delay rotary control adjusts the alarm delay from 1 to 60 seconds.

AC on/off is a toggle switch that activates AC power to the ventilator and internal battery charger.

Run on/off is a toggle switch that activates power to the motor.

Patient/Operator Safeguards

Alarms. *I:E ratio alarm* — a red light warns of potential machine breath error. *Low pressure alarm* — an audible alarm with a red light that warns of low circuit pressure below alarm limit. *High pressure limit* has both audible and red light systems that warn the operator that pressure in the system has reached the high-pressure alarm limit. When *AC power* is on, a *blue light* will be on. When *power is activated to the motor, a green light* will be on. A *red light* indicates a *power switchover* to the *internal battery*. If an *external battery* is used, an *amber light* will indicate that the ventilator is operating on the external battery. A *white light warns* of a *low battery,* either *internal or external.*

Power Sources. 120 AC, 60 Hz, 12 DC external battery (up to 30 hours), internal battery (up to 3 hours).

Optional Accessories

Oxygen accumulator, cascade humidifier, cover for faceplate, patient call switch, 6 feet or 12 feet of external battery cable.

Thompson GS Ventilator

The Thompson GS is a small portable ventilator placed in a sturdy suitcase that houses a powerful mechanism for ventilating a patient by tracheostomy, mouth, or pneumobelt. The ventilator can use AC or external 12-volt battery. By design this ventilator can be placed on the patient's wheelchair to provide maximum patient mobility.

Specifications

Rates from 6 to 24 breaths per minute
Pressure range from 15 to 45 cmH$_2$O
Sigh pressures of 30 to 45 cmH$_2$O, rates of 4 to 6 sigh breaths
per hour (These sigh breaths can be set automatically for
12 to 14 seconds, or manually.)

Patient/Operator Safeguards

Alarms. A patient-operated call alarm that works with the ventilator on or off. Low-pressure alarm and light, fail to cycle alarm and light, power failure alarm that will work on AC and DC power, and an alarm delay switch good for 30 to 90 seconds.

Power Source.   120 volts, 60 Hz, and 12-volt external battery.

Optional Accessories

Cascade humidifier, patient call switch, and battery cables.

Bear 33 Home Care Ventilator

The Bear 33 is said to be easier to use than any other ventilator on the market at this time. The ventilator is portable and can be powered by 120-AC, 60-Hz, an internal 12-DC or an external battery 12-DC system. While the unit is connected to an AC power source the ventilator will charge both the internal and external batteries. The panel controls are digital, so all information is easy to find and read. A test button allows a quick check of displays and integrity of LCDs. Tamper-proof panel lock and sealed splash-proof panel will prevent accidental or unwanted changes in ventilator functions. The Bear Company has an extensive patient/hospital training program, making use of the Bear 33 very easy to learn.

Controls

All controls are touch button. Control, assist/control, SIMV modes, tidal volumes 100 to 2200 ml, respiratory rates of 2.0 to 40 breaths/minute, peak flows 20 to 120 L/minute, and sigh breath at one and a half times the tidal volume.

Alarms

High pressure set from 0 to 80 cmH$_2$O, low pressure set from 3 to 70 cmH$_2$O, apnea alarm, low battery, power charge, ventilator inoperative, and complete power failure.

Puritan-Bennett 2800 Portable Ventilator

The Puritan-Bennett 2800 portable volume ventilator is an electrically powered, microprocessor-controlled ventilator designed for a wide range of patient applications. The ventilator can be powered by either 120-AC, external 12-DC, or internal 12-DC systems.

Controls

A five-position rotary control provides power-off, charge internal battery, control, assist, and SIMV modes. Tidal volumes are adjustable from 50 to 2800 ml, normal sigh volume setting above tidal volume 125 to 2800 ml, rates adjustable from 1 to 69 breaths/minute, and peak flows from 40 to 125 L/minute.

Alarms

An audible and visual alarm for intense I : E ratio of 1 : 0.8 or less or if delivered breath rate is less than set breaths per minute, low-pressure alarm from 2 to 32 cmH_2O, high-pressure alarm from 10 to 70 cmH_2O, apnea alarm during SIMV set at 15 seconds, low battery, power switchover, and ventilator malfunction alarms.

TROUBLESHOOTING HOME VENTILATORS

In most cases, trouble shooting a home ventilator is the same as any other ventilator, but with a few exceptions.

Problems and Possible Causes

Problem.   Alarm sounds as soon as the unit is turned on?

Probable Cause.   Low-pressure alarm sounds until the first breath that exceeds low-pressure setting is pumped.

Problem.   Alarm sounds as soon as the unit is turned on, but unit does not operate?

Probable Cause.   DC fuse blown. Check and replace. Some units have circuit breakers. Reset by pushing in button.

Problem.   Alarm sounds softly at peak pressure of each breath and increases in volume as use continues?

Probable Cause. Low-voltage alarm begins sounding when battery reaches low charge level. Connect AC power cord.

Problem. Green light or *on* light does not glow when unit is connected to 110-volt outlet?

Probable Cause. AC fuse blown. Check and replace. Or AC power cord not properly connected. Check cord.

Problem. Green light or *on* light blinks slightly?

Probable Cause. This is a normal operation and occurs when the batteries are fully charged.

Problem. Orange or red light does not glow, unit operates, no AC power?

Probable Cause. Indicator lamp defective. Replace. If green lamp is defective it will affect operation of red and orange lamps.

Problem. With external battery connected, no AC power, red lamp glows brightly, unit will not operate, clicking sound can be heard inside unit?

Probable Cause. External battery incorrectly connected. Check wiring instructions.

Problem. With external battery connected, no AC power, unit operates with red lamp glowing?

Probable Cause. Unit is not switching to external battery. Check DC power cord connections.

Problem. After extended use on external battery, orange and red lights both blink, clicking noises, and erratic operation?

Probable Cause. External battery is low. Unit is attempting to switch to internal battery.

Problem. After extended use of batteries, unit is connected to AC power, green light blinks brightly, and clicking is heard?

Probable Cause. Battery is at a very low charge level. Clicking is caused by an automatic circuit breaker that opens when charge current is too high. As battery reaches higher charge level, breaker will remain closed. To prevent this, recharge more often or use a heavier battery.

HOME CARE TRAINING CHECKLIST

A home training checklist, completed before the patient goes home, can aid in the relief of most problems that could happen later. The therapist or home care provider should instruct the patient and family on the use of the ventilator and allow for "practice" before the patient goes home.

The following is a sample of the home care training checklist:

1. Can give brief description of dials when used.
2. Follows flow of air through tubes.
3. Can trouble shoot high and low alarms.
4. Can use a hand resuscitator.
5. Can use a respirometer.
6. Can use O_2 analyzer.
7. Can clean circuits.
8. Can operate and maintain nebulizer.
9. Handwashing technique.
10. Suctioning equipment.
11. Suctioning procedure.
12. Tracheostomy care, stoma care, tracheostomy tube change, cuff inhalation.
13. Emergency procedures (cardiopulmonary resuscitation)
14. Knows what to do if power failure happens.
15. Knows what to do if equipment failure happens.
16. Knows early warning signs, color changes, swelling, changes in behavior, and changes in respiratory rate.
17. Home environmental needs, restriction on visitors and children, and *no smoking*.

VENTILATOR MAINTENANCE

Procedure

1. Always wash your hands before working with the ventilator.

2. Suction patient.

3. Manual ventilator should always be kept close by and in good working order.

4. Periodically, check the tubing for condensation and drain water into a water trap or wastepaper can.

5. Routinely check water level in the cascade humidifier.

6. Before changing the ventilator circuit, have a clean circuit assembled and ready to use. During the procedure, the patient can be hand ventilated or if there is a second ventilator the patient can be placed on this unit while tubing is being changed. However, if the patient has only one unit and no one is available to hand ventilate the patient for you, the patient may be able to ventilate himself with a hand resuscitator.

7. Fill a clean cascade humidifier with sterile water.

8. Bypass the humidifier by placing the patient circuit directly on the output side of the ventilator.

9. Disconnect the dirty cascade from the ventilator and replace with a clean cascade.

10. Place clean circuit on the output side of the cascade humidifier.

11. Place a clean wide-bore tube to the inlet side of the cascade.

12. Inform the patient that you are going to change to a new circuit, disconnect the patient from the unit and remove old circuit, and connect the clean tubing.

13. Before placing the circuit back on the patient, check the circuit for leaks by placing a clean gauze over the patient connector and cycling the ventilator.

14. Place the patient back on the ventilator and check to see that patient's chest and manometer both rise on the next inspiration.

15. *If* step 14 fails, hand ventilate until the problem can be corrected.

CLEANING VENTILATOR TUBING

Proper cleaning is of the utmost importance to help minimize the possibility of infection from using contaminated equipment. Frequency for cleaning should be every day to every other day, depending on equipment used; this can vary from company to company.

Procedure

1. Disassemble the humidifier and tubing.
2. Wash the parts using warm soapy water.
3. Thoroughly rinse the parts and shake off excess water.
4. Disinfect the equipment using the following method:
   a. Soak for 10 minutes in Quatimine A or a similar cleaner.
   b. Rinse well (you may need to use a rinse solution, if required by manufacturer).
   c. If using A-33 Dry solution/Instasan, keep in a covered container and away from heat.
5. Shake excess water from parts and dry in a clean place.

Follow the manufacturer's requirements for cleaning; the above is only a guide.

CLEANING SUCTION EQUIPMENT

Suction equipment should be cleaned every day. The secretion bottle may need to be emptied more often. The following is a guide for cleaning suction equipment.

Procedure

1. Disassemble and wash vacuum bottle with lid, connection tubing, and suction tip in hot soapy water, and rinse.

2. Dry bottle, lid, and tip with dry towel. Shake or blow dry connecting tubing.

3. Reassemble equipment.

4. Be sure lid is dry; no moisture should get into connecting tubing.

5. If moisture gets into cylinder, disassemble, wash, and dry.

MANUAL VENTILATORS

A manual ventilator is a bag-value device used to deliver a volume of air to the patient. Normally, the patient valve connects directly onto the patient's tracheostomy tube. In the event the patient does not have a tracheostomy tube, the bag can be equipped with a face mask for ventilation.

By squeezing the bag, air is pushed out of the bag through the patient valve into the lungs. When the bag is released the air from the patient exits through the patient valve and into room air, while at the same time fresh air enters the bag through the check valve at the end of the bag.

Procedure for Manual Ventilation

1. Connect the manual ventilator to the tracheostomy tube. Make sure the oxygen is turned on.

2. If the patient breathes on his own, squeeze the bag as he begins to inhale. If the patient does not breathe on his own, begin squeezing as soon as the bag is connected.

3. Observe the patient's chest while ventilating. Be sure the chest rises.

4. Release the bag after an observable rise in the chest.

5. Ventilate at a rate of 10 to 14 breaths per minute, or at the same rate as the patient's ventilator.

6. If the patient's chest does not rise and a resistance is felt, you must check the patient's breath sounds. If there is no air movement, you can try to insert a suction tube and suction the patient; if you cannot pass the suction tube, replace the tracheostomy tube.

TRACHEOSTOMY CLEANING FOR THE HOME CARE PATIENT

Tracheostomy cleaning will help prevent the buildup of mucus in the airway, which could cause a restriction to breathing.

The equipment needed to care for the tracheostomy tube includes hydrogen peroxide, sterile water, two small basins, and a soft nonabrasive brush or pipe cleaner.

Procedure for Tracheostomy Cleaning

1. Wash hands.
2. Suction and hand-ventilate the patient.
3. If the patient is ventilator-dependent, secure a second inner cannula and place the patient back on the ventilator.
4. Mix the hydrogen peroxide and sterile water in one basin at a 1:1 ratio.
5. Place the inner cannula into the hydrogen peroxide. Let it soak while you clean around the stoma.
6. Gently clean the inner cannula with the brush or pipe cleaner.
7. Rinse the inner cannula in sterile water, using the second basin.
8. Shake off excess water and replace inner cannula.

Procedure for Stoma Care

1. Remove the old tracheostomy dressing.
2. Clean stoma site using peroxide and cotton swabs, and rinse with sterile water. Dry site with 4 × 4 gauze sponges.
3. Fold 4 × 4 gauze for dressing.
4. If tracheostomy ties are dirty, change them at this time.
5. Stabilize the tube while cleaning and replace the dressing.

HOME CARE AEROSOL THERAPY

Aerosol therapy is used in the home as an aid to bronchial hygiene. Small hand-held nebulizers are the most economical means of delivery of inhaled medications. This type of device is preferred over IPPB if the patient has an adequate inspiratory capacity.

The goals of aerosol therapy include:

To restore and maintain the mucus blanket

To hydrate dried, retained secretions

To promote expectoration and deliver medications

Although IPPB has been the subject of much controversy,

under certain circumstances it does have a place in pulmonary rehabilitation. Many pulmonary patients have had home IPPB units for years and are psychologically dependent on their use. To take away these units would be an injustice to these patients. Although IPPB should never be solely used as a means to deliver medications, it can be of use in aiding the delivery of medications to patients who are unable to perform an adequate inspiratory capacity.

The goals of IPPB are:

To improve and promote the cough mechanism

To improve distribution of ventilation

To deliver medications (only if no other means can safely and conveniently deliver the medication)

CHEST PHYSICAL THERAPY

Chest physical therapy (CPT) can be a very effective aid in the removal of accumulated secretions. The patient and his family should be instructed in its delivery and encouraged to perform CPT at home. Figures 6–1 to 6–9 show the body

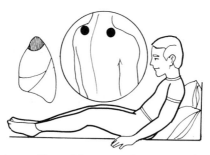

Figure 6–1. Upper lobes—apical segment: client should be placed in a sitting position on a bed, or this position may be done while the client is in a chair. The client should lean back on a pillow at approximately a 30-degree angle. Clapping is done over the area between the clavicle and the top of the scapula on each side. (From Saperstein, AB and Frazier, MA: Introduction to Nursing Practice. FA Davis, Philadelphia, 1980, p 694, with permission.)

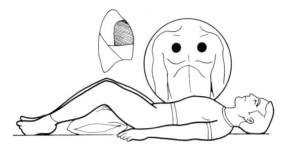

Figure 6 – 2. Upper lobes — anterior segment: the client is in a flat position on his back with a pillow placed under the knees. Percussion is done between the clavicle and the nipple on each side of the chest. (From Saperstein, AB and Frazier, MA: Introduction to Nursing Practice. FA Davis, Philadelphia, 1980, p 694, with permission.)

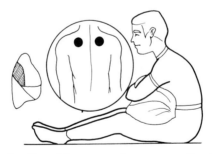

Figure 6 – 3. Upper lobes — posterior segments: client is placed in a sitting position and leans forward over a folded pillow. Percussion is done over the upper back on each side of the chest. (From Saperstein, AB and Frazier, MA: Introduction to Nursing Practice. FA Davis, Philadelphia, 1980, p 694, with permission.)

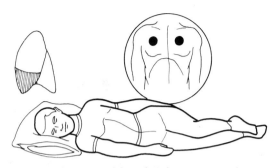

Figure 6–4. Left upper lobe—lingular segments: client lies on right side at a 45-degree angle. Pillows may be placed behind the shoulder and hips. Knees should be flexed. Percussion is done over the nipple area. (From Saperstein, AB and Frazier, MA: Introduction to Nursing Practice. FA Davis, Philadelphia, 1980, p 694, with permission.)

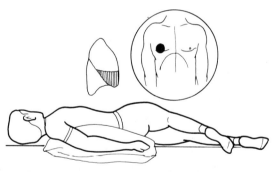

Figure 6–5. Right middle lobe—lateral and medial segments: client has head down on the left side and rotates body at 45-degree angle. Pillows may be placed behind the client at the shoulder and hip. Percussion is done over the nipple area. (From Saperstein, AB and Frazier, MA: Introduction to Nursing Practice. FA Davis, Philadelphia, 1980, p 694, with permission.)

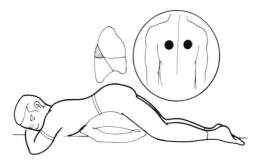

Figure 6–6. Lower lobe—superior segment: client lies flat on abdomen. Pillows are placed under the hips. Percussion is done over the middle third of the back (below scapula and on either side of the spine). (From Saperstein, AB and Frazier, MA: Introduction to Nursing Practice. FA Davis, Philadelphia, 1980, p 694, with permission.)

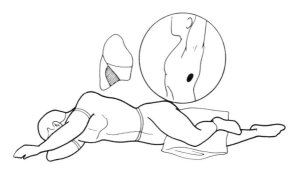

Figure 6–7. Lower lobes—anterior basal segment: provision is made to elevate the foot of the bed about 30 degrees. The client lies on side with head down and a pillow under the knees. Percussion is done over the lower ribs beneath the axilla. (From Saperstein, AB and Frazier, MA: Introduction to Nursing Practice. FA Davis, Philadelphia, 1980, p 695, with permission.)

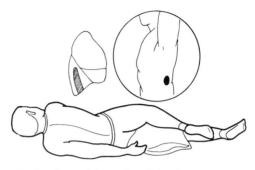

Figure 6–8. Lower lobes—lateral basal segment: provision is made to elevate the foot of the bed about 30 degrees. The client lies on the abdomen and rotates the body about 45 degrees. The upper leg may be flexed and supported over a pillow. Percussion is done over the uppermost part of the lower ribs. (From Saperstein, AB and Frazier, MA: Introduction to Nursing Practice. FA Davis, Philadelphia, 1980, p 695, with permission.)

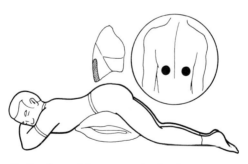

Figure 6–9. Lower lobes—posterior basal segment: provision is made to elevate the foot of the bed about 30 degrees. The client lies on his abdomen with the head down with a pillow under the hips. Percussion is done over the lower ribs close to the spine on each side of the posterior chest. (From Saperstein, AB and Frazier, MA: Introduction to Nursing Practice. FA Davis, Philadelphia, 1980, p 695, with permission.)

positions the patient should assume during CPT and will help you instruct these patients.

BIBLIOGRAPHY

The works listed below are also suggested readings that will give the reader more information concerning the chapter content.

Abels, LF: Mosby's Manual of Critical Care. CV Mosby, St. Louis, 1979.

Monroe, R: Handbook of Home Care. Mountaineer Medical Services, Charleston, 1986.

O'Ryan, JA: Pulmonary Rehabilitation from Hospital to Home. Year Book Medical Publishers, Chicago, 1984.

Saperstein, AB and Frazier, MA: Introduction to Nursing Practice. FA Davis, Philadelphia, 1980.

NOTES

Neonatal and Pediatric Respiratory Care

Neonatal and pediatric care has become one of the fastest growing areas in respiratory care. We must remember that we are not dealing with full-grown adults. Changes occur faster with infants and children and we must keep a close watch for these changes. Studies have shown that an infant does feel pain and we should not lose the caring side of our feelings by forgetting this. The key to neonatal and pediatric care is fast recognition of changing clinical signs with a fast but gentle response to these changes.

NEONATAL AND
PEDIATRIC DISEASES

Aspiration

There are two forms of neonatal aspiration: meconium aspiration and aspiration of amniotic or vaginal substances.

Possible Causes

Aspiration may occur before birth. Causes may be premature placental separation, ingested amniotic fluid, cervical mucus, or meconium, and postmature infants.

Clinical Findings

Chest x-rays show patchy densities, flattened diaphragms, wide-spaced ribs. The infant may have respiratory distress, tachypnea, grunting, retractions, rales, low Apgar scores. Skin may be dry and scaly. Nailbeds may be yellow-green as a result of intrauterine meconium aspiration.

Treatment

Pharyngeal suctioning as soon as the head is delivered, then tracheal suctioning should be done under direct visualization of the chords immediately after birth. Humidified oxygen, thermoregulation, ventilatory assistance only after suctioning, and removal of swallowed meconium from the stomach.

Bronchopulmonary Dysplasia (BPD)

BPD is caused by high oxygen concentration and/or positive-pressure ventilation. Onset is usually after 10 to 20 days following the start of oxygen therapy.

Clinical Findings

The patient will have CO_2 retention with a history of receiving high FI_{O_2} and mechanical ventilation. The chest x-ray may show fine granular densities, small, round, lucent area, irregular densities, atelectasis, thick mucus, and lung fibrosis with flattened diaphragms. Pulmonary hypertension, cor pulmonale, and heart failure are common findings.

Treatment

Prevention is the best treatment. The use of low peak pressure with PEEP and low FI_{O_2} for shorter time periods will help reduce the incidence of BPD. For infants who do get BPD, treatment should include high humidity, chest physical therapy, and suctioning.

Hyaline Membrane Disease (HMD or RDS)

The principal factor in HMD is a deficiency in the surfactant production in the lungs. It is primarily found in premature or low-birth-weight infants and infants of diabetic mothers.

Clinical Findings

The infant will show signs of tachypnea or bradypnea (in severely depressed infants), nasal flaring with grunting, cyanosis, retractions with decreased breath sounds, and very decreased muscle tone. X-rays show a ground-glass appearance; arterial blood gases show acidosis, hypoxia, and hypercapnia.

Treatment

Supportive oxygen therapy and CPAP can be used to establish FRC, decrease atelectasis, and decrease the work of breathing.

Pneumothorax

Pneumothorax may result from the high distending pressures needed to open unexpanded lungs at birth.

Clinical Findings

The patient may show signs of cyanosis, tachypnea, grunting, nasal flaring, possible tracheal shift, and a shift of the apical pulse.

Treatment

When infants are in distress a physician should do a needle evacuation or chest tube insertion to relieve the pneumothorax. These infants should be on oxygen, at a FI_{O_2} high enough to help correct any hypoxia. For infants who are asymptomatic, watch heart rate, respiratory rate, and color, and have frequent chest films done, watching for any enlargement of the pneumothorax.

Cystic Fibrosis

Cystic fibrosis is a hereditary disease occurring in 1 of 1500 to 2500 births. It is a recessive hereditary disease.

Clinical Findings

These patients have a high concentration of sweat electrolytes (chlorides). Sweat test of over 60 mEq/L is a common finding. Abnormal mucus secretion and elimination are the most common problems found in the cystic fibrosis patient. Pulmonary secretions are viscid, which blocks small bronchi and bronchioles. *Pseudomonas aeruginosa* and *Staphylococcus aureus* are also common findings in these patients. Patients develop bronchitis, bronchiectasis, bronchiolitis, atelectasis, abscess formation, and pneumonia. X-rays show atelectasis, fibrosis, diffuse hyperinflation (air trapping), and increased lung markings with flat diaphragms. Pulmonary function tests show a decreased vital capacity, decreased peak flow, increased airway resistance, and a decreased maximum voluntary ventilation.

Respiratory Treatment

Removal of secretions and control of infections are of primary concern. The treatment most used today consists of high-humidity devices, bronchodilators, mucolytics, postural drainage, vibration, and clapping with breathing exercises, although there is a move currently toward treating the disease through increased vitamin intake in the patient's diet.

Respiratory Distress in the Newborn Infant

Possible Causes

Respiratory distress in the newborn infant may result from respiratory distress syndrome, transient tachypnea, meconium aspiration, pneumothorax, hypovolemia, anemia, polycythemia, persistent fetal circulation, and congestive heart failure. These are only the more common forms of respiratory distress seen in the newborn infant.

Clinical Findings

The respiratory rate is greater than 60 breaths/minute. There are cyanosis, grunting, nasal flaring, retractions, and tachypnea.

Treatment

Administer emergency therapy. This therapy depends on the severity of the symptoms. FI_{O_2} should be kept at the lowest setting in order to keep a Pa_{O_2} between 50 to 70 mmHg. It should also be kept in mind that in an infant cyanosis may reflect a Pa_{O_2} of 32 to 42 mmHg, so an early and vigorous intervention to establish the etiology is of the utmost importance. Possible ventilatory support and/or PEEP/CPAP therapy may be used in moderate and severe cases.

Epiglottitis

Possible Causes

Epiglottitis occurs mostly in children 2 to 6 years of age, although it has been reported in an infant 8 days old. It is more common in males than in females. It is usually caused by *Hemophilus influenzae* type B and is more often isolated in the blood than in epiglottic or pharyngeal swabs. Also, *Streptococcus viridans*, *Staphylococcus aureus*, and group A β-hemolytic streptococci have been reported to cause epiglottitis.

Clinical Findings

There is a history of sudden onset of sore throat, increasing pain, lethargy, and fever. As edema worsens, the patient will assume a classic position of sitting up, and leaning forward with the neck slightly extended. The tongue may protrude, with saliva drooling from the mouth. There is inspiratory and expiratory stridor with intercostal retractions. A cough may be present but is very rarely croupy. Temperature is usually greater than 38.5° C. Leukocytosis greater than $15,000/\mu L$ with a left shift and lateral neck x-ray showing swelling of the soft tissues are also common findings.

Treatment

Treatment has been the subject of debate. The prevailing opinion is in favor of nasotracheal intubation rather than tracheostomy. A skilled physician should be on hand to intubate the patient, and this should be done if possible in the operating room with equipment for an emergency tracheotomy present. Tube size used should be one to two sizes smaller than usually inserted. Vigorous hydration and antibiotics are the mainstay of therapy. Ampicillin, 200 to 400 mg/kg/day by IV in four divided doses, and chloramphenicol, 100 mg/kg/day in four divided doses, are recommended. Once antibiotic sensitivities of the blood cultures become available, adjustments can be made, if needed, in antibiotic therapy. The use of nebulized racemic epinephrine has not been studied, and *it may even cause complete upper airway obstruction.*

Croup, Laryngotracheobronchitis (LTB)

Possible Causes

LTB occurs in children and infants 3 months to 3 years old. Twice as many males as females are affected and it may be seasonal in nature. Respiratory syncytial virus, parainfluenza virus types 2 and 3 and types A and B are the more common causes of croup.

Clinical Findings

LTB seen in the fall and early winter is caused by parainfluenza virus and in the mid winter and early spring by syncytial virus. It has a gradual onset from 1 to 7 days, low-grade fever usually below 38°C, hoarseness, and a "seal bark" cough with inspiratory stridor and retractions. Anteroposterior and lateral neck x-rays show what is known as "steeple sign," which is a narrowing of the trachea, a classic radiologic finding of LTB.

Treatment

Treatment consists of humidification (cool mist), hydration, and oxygenation. FI_{O_2} of 30% to 40% with face mask or croup tent, using high humidity, is effective therapy. The use of epinephrine should be limited to inpatients, because of possible rebound edema. In rare cases, nasotracheal intubation may be necessary and for a duration of hospitalization of 1 to 2 weeks.

NORMAL LAB VALUES FOR INFANTS

Table 7–1 lists the normal lab values for infants.

NEONATAL AND PEDIATRIC VENTILATORS

Babybird 2A

The Babybird 2A ventilator is an electronically controlled, pneumatically powered, time-cycled, pressure-limited, and continuous-flow ventilator.

Modes

CMV (controlled mechanical ventilation)
IMV (intermittent mandatory ventilation)
CPAP (continuous positive airway pressure)

Parameters

Inspiratory time, 0.4 to 2.5 sec
Expiratory time, 0.4 to 10 sec
Cycling frequency, off to 120 BPM
Peak inspiratory pressure, 0 to 80 $cmH_2O \pm 10\%$ at 10 L/minute
Flow rate, 0 to 30 L/minute $\pm 10\%$

Alarms

Visual and audible alarms include:
Source pressure low preset at 38 psig
Incompatible timer setting preset at 0.2 sec expiratory time
Power failure

Sechrist

The Sechrist ventilator is a time-cycled, pressure-limited, pneumatically powered, fluidic, and electronically controlled ventilator.

Modes

CMV (controlled mechanical ventilation)

Table 7-1. NORMAL LAB VALUES FOR INFANTS

Age	Hemoglobin (g/dl)	RBC (10⁶/μL)	Hematocrit (%)
Cord blood	14.6 – 19.6	5.4	56.6
day 1	21.2 (18.2)	5.6 (4.7)	56.1
1 week	19.6 (16.3)	5.3 (4.4)	52.7
2 weeks	18.0 (14.5)	5.1 (4.1)	49.6
3 weeks	16.6 (12.9)	4.9 (3.7)	46.6
1 month	15.6 (10.9)	4.7 (3.2)	44.6

Age	Activated PTT (sec)	PT (sec)	TT (sec)
Preterm infant			
31 weeks (cord blood)	105	15 – 22	15 – 20
48 weeks	75	15 – 22	15 – 20
Full-term infant (cord blood)	70	12 – 17	10 – 20
48 hours	60	12 – 20	10 – 16
Child	30 – 40	10 – 12	10 – 15

Test	Age	Value
SGOT	Birth to 1 month	0 – 67 IU/L
SGPT	Birth to 1 month	0 – 54 IU/L
Alkaline phosphatase	Birth to 1 month	20 – 225 IU/L
	1 month to 3 months	73 – 226 IU/L

CPK		
Premature	0–100 U/L
Birth to 3 weeks	30–100 U/L
3 months	15–50 U/L

LDH	
Birth to 1 week	150–590
1 month	185–404
2 years	110–244

Age	WBC	Neutrophils	Eosinophils	Basophils	Lymphocytes	Monocytes
Birth	9.0–30.0	6.0–26.0	20–850	0–649	2.0–11.0	0.4–3.1
1 week	5.0–21.0	1.5–10.0	70–1100	0–250	2.0–17.0	0.3–2.7
2 weeks	5.0–20.0	1.0–9.5	70–1000	0–230	2.0–17.0	0.2–2.4

Bilirubin Direct   0.1 mg/dl
Bilirubin Total   0.3–1.3 mg/dl

	Premature	Full-term
Cord	<2 mg/dl	<2 mg/dl
0–1 day	<8 mg/dl	<6 mg/dl
1–2 days	<12 mg/dl	<8 mg/dl
3–5 days	<16 mg/dl	<12 mg/dl

(continued)

Table 7-1 — *Continued*

Glucose (FBS)	Normal Value
Premature infant	20–60 mg/dl
Newborn	30–80 mg/dl
Child	60–100 mg/dl
Thereafter	70–110 mg/dl

Serum Electrolytes

Potassium (K^+)	3.5–5.3 mEq/L
Sodium (Na^+)	136–145 mEq/L
Chloride (Cl^-)	96–108 mEq/L
Bicarbonate (HCO_3^-)	22–30 mEq/L
Phosphate (PO_4)	
Newborn	4–10.5 mg/dl
1 year	4–6.8 mg/dl
5 years	3.6–6.5 mg/dl
Calcium (Ca^{++}) (total)	
Premature	6–10 mg/dl
Full-term	7–12 mg/dl
Children	8–11 mg/dl
Magnesium (MG^{++})	

Newborn	1.52–2.33 mEq/L
Children	1.40–1.90 mEq/L

Serum Enzymes

Alkaline phosphate

Newborn	20–266 IU/ml
1 month	50–260 IU/ml
7–10 years	45–273 IU/ml

Acid phosphate

Newborn	7.4–19.4 IU/ml
2–13 years	6.4–152 IU/ml
Amylase	60–160 somogyi units/dl

Miscellaneous

Sweat Test
Sodium
10–80 mEq/L

Chloride
4–60 mEq/L

Urine
pH, 5.00–7.00
Glucose and acetone, negative
Specific gravity in the newborn, 1.00–1.020

IMV (intermittent mandatory ventilation)
CPAP (continuous positive airway pressure)

Parameters

Inspiratory time, 0.1 to 2.9 sec
Expiratory time, 0.3 to 60 sec
I : E ratio, 10 : 1 to 1 : 600 (read out 1 : 0.1 to 1 : 99)
Rate, 1 to 150 BPM
Inspiratory pressure, 7 to 70 cmH$_2$O
Expiratory pressure, −2 to 15 cmH$_2$O

Alarms

Audible and visual alarms include low airway pressure, leaks, patient disconnect, fail to cycle, source gas failure, power failure, apnea, and prolonged inspiration. This ventilator has a manual test to check microprocessor function, displays, and alarm functions.

Bear Cub

The Bear Cub ventilator is an electrically and pneumatically powered, electronically controlled, single-circuit with continuous flow ventilator.

Modes

CPAP
CMV/IMV

Parameters

Pressure limit, adjustable from 0 to 72 cmH$_2$O
Rate, 1 to 150 BPM
Inspiratory time, 0.1 to 3.0 sec
Flow rate, 3 to 30 L/minute
PEEP/CPAP, −2 to 20 cmH$_2$O

Alarms

There are alarms for low inspiratory pressure, low PEEP/CPAP, prolonged inspiratory pressure set for 3.5 sec, ventilator inoperative, and $I:E$ ratio.

Bourns BP 200

The Bourns BP 200 ventilator is an electrically and pneumatically powered, electronically controlled, single-circuit, continuous-flow ventilator.

Modes

CPAP
IPPB/IMV

Parameters

Rate, previous units 1 to 60 or 1 to 80 BPM; new units 1 to 150 BPM
$I:E$ ratio, $4:1$ to $1:10$
Maximum inspiratory time, 0.1 to 3.0 sec for new units, 0.1 to 5.0 sec for previous units
Flow rates, 0 to 20 L/minute
CPAP/PEEP, 0 to 20 cmH$_2$O
Pressure limit, 12 cmH$_2$O at 2 L/minute to 80 cmH$_2$O at 20 L/minute

Alarms

There are no true alarms, but indicators include power, insufficient expiratory time, and inspiratory limit indicator.

Healthdyne 105

The Healthdyne 105 ventilator is an electrically powered, pneumatically operated, microprocessor-controlled, single-circuit, continuous-flow ventilator.

Modes

IPPV/IMV
CPAP

Parameters

Rate, 1 to 150 BPM
Inspiratory time, 0.1 to 4.9 sec
Pressure limit, 1 to 70 cmH$_2$O
PEEP/CPAP, 0 to 20 cmH$_2$O
Flow rate, two controls—3 to 20 or 20 to 60 L/minute

Alarms

Low pressure, 1 to 100 cmH$_2$O
High pressure, 3 to 100 cmH$_2$O
Delay low pressure, 0 to 90 sec
Insufficient expiratory time, <0.2 sec
Inverse I:E ratio, >4:1
Power loss
System interrupt

PEDIATRIC CUFFLESS TRACHEOSTOMY TUBES

The dimensions of pediatric cuffless tracheostomy tubes are listed in Table 7–2.

SELECTION OF PEDIATRIC ENDOTRACHEAL TUBES

Table 7–3 lists the dimensions of endotracheal tubes for pediatric use.

DRUGS USED IN PEDIATRIC RESPIRATORY CARE

Tables 7–4 to 7–7 list the various drugs and their dosages used in neonatal and pediatric respiratory care.

Table 7-2. PEDIATRIC CUFFLESS
TRACHEOSTOMY TUBES

Jackson Size	Inner Diameter	Outer Diameter	Length
Shiley			
0	3.1	4.5	39
1	3.4	5.0	40
1.5	3.7	5.5	41
2	4.1	6.0	42
3	4.8	7.0	44
Portex			
0	3.0	4.5	41
1.5	3.8	5.0	46
3	4.5	6.0	52
3.5	5.3	7.0	55
4	6.0	8.0	59

Table 7-3. SELECTION OF
ENDOTRACHEAL TUBES

Weight or Age	Inner Diameter	French Size (Suction Catheter)	Length
<1000 g	2.5	6	8
>1000 g	3.0	6	9
Age 6 months	3.5	8	10
Age 1 year	4.0-4.5	8	12
Age 2 years	5.0-5.5	8	14
Age 2-4 years	5.5-6.0	10	15
Age 4-7 years	6.0-6.5	10	16
Age 7-10 years	6.5-7.0	10	17
Age 10-12 years	7.0-7.5	10	20

Table 7-4. DRUGS USED IN ACLS FOR INFANTS AND CHILDREN

Drug	Dose	How Supplied	Remarks
Atropine sulfate	0.01–0.03 mg/kg	0.1 mg/ml	...
Calcium chloride	0.3 ml/kg	(10%)	Give slowly
Dexamethasone sodium phosphate	0.3 mg/kg/24 hours	4 mg/ml	...
Dopamine hydrochloride	5–20 μg/kg/minute	40 mg/ml	α-Receptor dominate at ≥ 10 μg/kg/minute
Epinephrine	0.1 ml/kg	1:10,000	1:1000 must be diluted
Epinephrine infusion	Start at 0.1 μg/kg/minute	1:1000 (1 mg)	Usual effect ≤1.5 μg/kg/minute
Furosemide	1 mg/kg/dose	10 mg/ml	...
Isoproterenol hydrochloride	Start at 0.1 μg/kg/minute	1 mg/5 ml	Usual effect 0.1–1.0 μg/kg/minute

Lidocaine	1 mg/kg/dose	10 mg/ml (1%) 20 mg/ml (2%)	. . .
Lidocaine infusion	10–50 μg/kg/minute	10 mg/ml (1%) 20 mg/ml (2%) 40 mg/ml (4%)	. . .
Norepinephrine	Start at 0.1 μg/kg/minute	1 mg/ml	Titrate to desired effect
Naloxone hydrochloride	0.01 mg/kg/dose	0.4 mg/ml; 0.02 mg/ml	Short half-life
Sodium nitroprusside	Start at 0.5 μg/kg/minute	10 mg/ml	Usual effect at 1–10 μg/kg/minute
Sodium bicarbonate	1–2 mEq/kg/dose or 0.3 × kg × base deficit	1 mEq/ml	Should be diluted in newborns

(From McIntyre, JD: Textbook of Advanced Cardiac Life Support. American Heart Association, Dallas, 1983, with permission.)

Table 7–5. EPINEPHRINE* INFUSION CHART FOR INFANTS AND CHILDREN

Dilution A: 0.5 mg (0.5 ml 1:1000) epinephrine in 100.0 ml 5% dextrose in water = 5 μg/ml
Dilution B: 1.0 mg (1.0 ml 1:1000) epinephrine in 100.0 ml 5% dextrose in water = 10 μg/ml
Dilution C: 2.0 mg (2.0 ml 1:1000) epinephrine in 100.0 ml 5% dextrose in water = 20 μg/ml
Dilution D: 4.0 mg (4.0 ml 1:1000) epinephrine in 100.0 ml 5% dextrose in water = 40 μg/ml

Weight (kg)	Dilution	Delivered Dose 0.1 μg/kg/minute Infusion Rate ml/hour	Dilution	Delivered Dose 0.5 μg/kg/minute Infusion Rate ml/hour
1	A	1	B	3
2	A	2	B	6
3	A	4	B	9
4	A	5	B	12
5	A	6	C	8
7	A	8	C	11
10	A	12	C	15

11	B	7	C	17
13	B	8	C	20
15	B	9	C	23
17	B	10	C	26
19	B	11	C	29
20	B	12	D	15
25	B	15	D	19
30	B	18	D	23
35	B	21	D	26
40	C	12	D	30

All calculations are rounded to the nearest full number.

Example: To infuse 0.5 μg/kg/minute to 7-kg infant: Prepare solution C by mixing 2.0 ml 1:1000 epinephrine in 100 ml 5% dextrose in water. Infuse at 11 ml/hour.

Caution: Epinephrine can cause tachycardia and dysrhythmias, especially at doses higher than 0.5 μg/kg/minute. Doses should be increased slowly in increments of 0.1 μg/kg/minute while the patient is carefully monitored.

(From McIntyre, JD: Textbook of Advanced Cardiac Life Support. American Heart Association, Dallas, 1983, with permission.)

Table 7-6. ISOPROTERENOL* INFUSION CHART FOR INFANTS AND CHILDREN

Dilution A: 0.5 mg (2.5 ml) isoproterenol in 97.5 ml 5% dextrose in water = 5 μg/ml
Dilution B: 1.0 mg (5.0 ml) isoproterenol in 95 ml 5% dextrose in water = 10 μg/ml
Dilution C: 2.0 mg (10 ml) isoproterenol in 90 ml 5% dextrose in water = 20 μg/ml
Dilution D: 4.0 mg (20 ml) isoproterenol in 80 ml 5% dextrose in water = 40 μg/ml

Weight (kg)	Delivered Dose 0.1 μg/kg/minute		Delivered Dose 0.5 μg/kg/minute	
	Dilution	Infusion Rate ml/hour	Dilution	Infusion Rate ml/hour
1	A	1	B	3
2	A	2	B	6
3	A	4	B	9
4	A	5	B	12
5	A	6	C	8
7	A	8	C	11
10	A	12	C	15

11	B	7	C	17
13	B	8	C	20
15	B	9	C	23
17	B	10	C	26
19	B	11	C	29
20	B	12	D	15
25	B	15	D	19
30	B	18	D	23
35	B	21	D	26
40	C	12	D	30

All calculations are rounded to the nearest full number.

Example: To infuse 0.5 μg/kg/minute to 4-kg infant: Prepare solution B by mixing 1.0 mg (5.0 ml) isoproterenol in 95 ml 5% dextrose in water. Infuse at 12 ml/hour.

Caution: Isoproterenol can cause tachycardia and dysrhythmias, especially at doses higher than 0.5 μg/kg/minute. Doses should be increased slowly in increments of 0.1 μg/kg/minute while the patient is carefully monitored.

(From McIntyre, JD: Textbook of Advanced Cardiac Life Support. American Heart Association, Dallas, 1983, with permission.)

Table 7-7. DOPAMINE INFUSION CHART FOR INFANTS AND CHILDREN

Dilution A: 100 mg dopamine in 500 ml 5% dextrose in water = 200 μg/ml
Dilution B: 200 mg in 500 ml 5% dextrose in water = 400 μg/ml
Dilution C: 400 mg in 500 ml 5% dextrose in water = 800 μg/ml

Weight (kg)	Dilution	Delivered Dose		
		5 μg/kg/minute	10 μg/kg/minute	15 μg/kg/minute
		Infusion rate ml/hour		
1	A	2	3	5
3	A	5	9	14
4	B	3	6	9
6	B	5	9	14
8	B	6	12	18

10	B	8	15	23
11	C	4	8	12
13	C	5	10	15
15	C	6	11	17
20	C	8	15	23
25	C	9	19	28
30	C	11	23	34
35	C	13	26	39
40	C	15	30	35

All calculations are rounded to the nearest full number.

Example: To infuse 10 μg/kg/minute to 6-kg infant: Prepare solution B by mixing 1 ampule of dopamine in 500 ml 5% dextrose in water. Infuse at 9 ml/hour.

(From McIntyre, JD: Textbook of Advanced Cardiac Life Support. American Heart Association, Dallas, 1983, with permission.)

BIBLIOGRAPHY

The works listed below are also suggested readings that will give the reader more information concerning the chapter content.

Abels, LF: Mosby's Manual of Critical Care. CV Mosby, St. Louis, 1979.

Byrne, CJ: Laboratory Tests. Addison-Wesley, Menlo Park, CA, 1986.

Daily, EK: Techniques in Bedside Hemodynamic Monitoring, ed 3. CV Mosby, St. Louis, 1985.

Kacmarck, RM: The Essentials of Respiratory Therapy, ed 2. Year Book Medical Publishers, Chicago, 1985.

McIntyre, JD: Textbook of Advanced Cardiac Life Support. American Heart Association, Dallas, 1983.

McPherson, SP: Respiratory Therapy Equipment, ed 3. CV Mosby, St. Louis, 1985.

Patterson, R: Current Drug Handbook. WB Saunders, Philadelphia, 1986.

Roberts, JT: Fundamentals of Tracheal Intubation. Grune & Stratton, New York, 1983.

NOTES

NOTES

8   **Respiratory Pharmacology***

Medications Often Used in Respiratory Care

Acetylcysteine (Mucomyst)
> Drug Type
> Drug Dose
> Remarks
> Hazards

Albuterol (Ventolin, Proventil)
> Drug Type
> Drug Dose
> Remarks
> Hazards

Aminophylline (Theophylline, Ethylenediamine)
> Drug Type
> Drug Dose
> Remarks
> Hazards

Beclomethasone Dipropionate (Vanceril)
> Drug Type
> Drug Dose
> Remarks
> Hazards

---

*The author and publisher have exerted every effort to ensure that drug selection and dosage set forth in this text are in accord with current recommendations and practice at the time of publication. The reader is urged to check the package insert for each drug for any change in indications and dosage and for added warnings and precautions.

Propranolol (Inderal)
>   Drug Type
>   Drug Dose
>   Remarks
>   Hazards

Sodium Bicarbonate
>   Drug Type
>   Drug Dose
>   Remarks
>   Hazards

Sodium Nitroprusside
>   Drug Type
>   Drug Dose
>   Remarks
>   Hazards

Drugs Used in Cardiac Arrest
Aerosol Antiviral Inhibitor
>   Virazole (Ribavirin)
>   Drug Type
>   Drug Dose
>   Remarks
>   Hazards

MEDICATIONS OFTEN USED IN RESPIRATORY CARE

Acetylcysteine (Mucomyst)

Drug Type

> Synthetic mucolytic

Drug Dose

> 10% or 20% dilute solution by inhalation; 3 to 5 ml of 10% or 20% tid or qid; 1 to 2 ml via endotracheal tube

Remarks

Used in bronchopulmonary disorders when mucolysis is desirable. This drug acts by breaking disulfide bonds of mucus, which decreases the thickness.

Hazards

Not to be used on asthmatic patients; may cause bronchospasm. Liquefied secretion must be removed by either suctioning or coughing.

Note that acetylcysteine may be given in the treatment of acetaminophen intoxication by oral administration. Loading dose of 140 mg/kg, then 50 mg/kg q4h for 17 doses. If vomiting occurs within 1 hour after dose, you can repeat that dose.

Albuterol (Ventolin, Proventil)

Drug Type

Synthetic sympathetic agent

Drug Dose

1 to 2 puffs q4 – 6h, which equals 90 μg

Remarks

For the relief of bronchospasm in patients with *reversible* obstructive lung disease. This drug is a selective β_2 bronchodilator. Improvement can occur within 15 minutes and can last 4 to 6 hours.

Hazards

Toxicity is possible if overused. Safety in children under the age of 12 years has not been established.

Aminophylline (Theophylline, Ethylenediamine)

Drug Type

Synthetic sympathomimetic

Drug Dose

5 to 7 mg/kg IV over 20 to 30 minutes, then 1.0 mg/kg/hour
    continuous IV
Cardiac or liver dysfunction: 0.25 mg/kg/hour
Neonates: 0.16 mg/kg/hour
Infants 2 to 6 months old: 0.5 mg/kg/hour
Infants 6 to 11 months old: 0.88 mg/kg/hour
Children: 1.0 mg/kg/hour
Oral dose: 20 to 28 mg/kg/day or 100 to 200 mg tid or qid

Remarks

Used in the relief of bronchial asthma, pulmonary emphysema, chronic bronchitis, and pulmonary edema, and may help
in patients with Cheyne-Stokes respirations. Works by relaxing
smooth muscle, stimulates the central nervous system, causes
diuresis, increases cardiac output. Metabolized by the liver.

Therapeutic serum levels are between 10 to 20 μg/ml;
levels above 20 μg/ml have toxic effects.

Hazards

Gastrointestinal irritation, nausea, vomiting, epigastric
pain, abdominal pain, headache, irritability, nervousness, dizziness, convulsions, transient palpitations, sinus tachycardia, and
increased pulse rate.

If cimetidine, erythromycin, IV furosemide, or influenza
vaccine has been given or congestive heart failure, liver disease,
or acute viral infection is present, these will decrease theophylline metabolism and increase risk of toxicity.

Beclomethasone Dipropionate (Vanceril)

Drug Type

Anti-inflammatory steroid

Drug Dose

50 μg dose/actuation, 12 to 16 inhalations/day or 3 to 4 inhalations qid
Children: no more than 10 inhalations/day

Remarks

For patients who require treatment with corticosteroids for the control of bronchial asthma symptoms

Hazards

Not indicated in asthma that can be controlled by bronchodilators, other nonsteroidal medication, patients who require steroids only infrequently, or in nonasthmatic bronchitis. Adrenal insufficiency following transfer to beclomethasone from systemic corticosteroids has resulted in death. The drug can suppress hypothalamic-pituitary-adrenal function.

Cromolyn Sodium (Intal)

Drug Type

Synthetic, prophylactic drug

Drug Dose

20 mg powder by inhalation qid or 20 mg in solution

Remarks

Adjunct therapy for the treatment of asthma. Inhibits the release of histamine and SRS-A. This drug is not an antihistamine, bronchodilator, or anti-inflammatory agent.

Hazards

Rash, cough, and bronchospasm may occur. Not to be used for acute asthma attacks, especially status asthmaticus.

Doxapram

Drug Type

Synthetic stimulant

Drug Dose

0.5 to 1.0 mg/lb IV; if given IM dose may be repeated.

Remarks

Stimulates respiration in patients with postanesthetic respiratory depression or apnea due to muscle-relaxant drugs. This drug stimulates all levels of the central nervous system.

Hazards

Contraindicated for patients with history of convulsions or those patients with incompetence of ventilatory mechanism due to muscle paresis, flail chest, pneumothorax, airway obstruction, extreme dyspnea, hypertension, and cardiovascular accidents. This drug is not recommended for children under the age of 12 years or during pregnancy.

Edrophonium Chloride (Tensilon)

Drug Type

Synthetic detoxifying agent

Drug Dose

Adults: 2 mg IV; 10 mg IV maximum dose for adults and pediatric patients >75 lb
Infants: 0.5 mg IV
Pediatric: <75 lb 1 mg IV; >75 lb 2 mg IV

Remarks

Anticurare agent used to terminate the action of curare. Also used in diagnosis of myasthenia gravis. Acts by displacing curare at the myoneural junction. Acts in 30 to 60 seconds and lasts for about 10 minutes.

The Tensilon Test. Give 1.0 mg IV; wait 60 seconds. If no improvement, give another 1.0 mg. If patient is myasthenic, clear respiratory improvement is noted. If the patient is in a cholinergic crisis, there will be an increase in secretions and respiratory deterioration.

Hazards

Rare side effects in therapeutic dosage. Some side effects are excess salivation, nausea, colic, and perspiration. Overdose may induce cholinergic crisis.

Ephedrine

Drug Type

Synthetic active ingredient of *Ephedra vulgaris* and *E. equisetina* (ma huang)

Drug Dose

15, 25, or 50 mg q3–4h orally or 3 mg/kg/day (divided into 4 to 6 doses); 25 to 50 mg q3–4h prn IM, IV, or 3% solution topically

Remarks

For hypotension, asthma, allergies, narcotic poisoning, also as a mydriatic, with neostigmine in myasthenia gravis and as a nasal decongestant. Stimulates both α- and β-adrenergic receptors. Causes the release of norepinephrine from presynaptic nerve terminals. Produces bronchodilation less intense but more prolonged than epinephrine.

Hazards

Headache, dizziness, palpitation, anxiety. Severe cases may cause cardiac depression, tremors, diaphoresis, and fainting.

Epinephrine, Racemic (Vaponefrin, Micronefrin)

Drug Type

Animal glands, natural sympathetic amine

Drug Dose

2.25% 1 : 8 ratio with saline to total of 2 to 3 ml q4 – 6h prn

Remarks

Symptomatic relief of bronchial asthma, anaphylactic, allergic, and other hypersensitivity reactions. This drug acts directly on both α- and β-adrenergic receptors.

Hazards

May cause burning, sneezing, rebound congestion, nasal dryness, tachycardia, palpitation, arrhythmias, nausea, and headache.

Isoetharine (Bronkosol)

Drug Type

Synthetic sympathetic amines

Drug Dose

0.25 to 0.5 ml 1.0% solution 1 : 3 ratio with saline q2 – 6h prn by aerosol

Remarks

Used for bronchodilation in bronchial asthma or reversible spasm. This drug is a β-adrenergic stimulant with little or no effect on α receptors. Rapidly absorbed with peak effect in 5 to 15 minutes and lasts up to 1 to 4 hours.

Hazards

Do not use with epinephrine. May produce changes in blood pressure and pulse. May cause palpitation, headache, dizziness, and nausea. Do not use drug if discolored (pink). Discourage excessive use. Must monitor heart rate in all patients, but more so in patients that may have hypertension, hyperthyroidism, or acute coronary disease.

Isoniazid (INH)

Drug Type

Synthetic antibacterial for tuberculosis

Drug Dose

50 to 200 mg tid or bid orally

Remarks

Used in the treatment of tuberculosis and also to prevent development of active tuberculosis in recently converted tuberculin-positive persons or people who may be high risk. INH is bacteriostatic to *Mycobacterium tuberculosis*.

Hazards

Peripheral neuritis is the most common side effect. Convulsions, optic neuritis, sedation, or incoordination may occur along with constipation, postural hypotension, dizziness, aplastic anemia, and elevated SGOT and SGPT. Severe hepatitis may occur. Patients who consume daily amounts of alcohol are at a higher risk and should be given aminosalicylic acid instead of INH.

Isoproterenol Hydrochloride (Isuprel)

Drug Type

Synthetic sympathetic agent

Drug Dose

10 to 15 mg orally, 0.25 to 0.50 ml/dose in 3 to 5 ml saline tid or qid aerosol 1 : 200 solution; pediatric 0.01 ml/kg/dose in 2 to 3 ml normal saline, not to exceed 0.3 ml/dose.

Remarks

A strong bronchodilator that facilitates expectoration of pulmonary secretions. Used for bronchial asthma, allergic conditions, congestion of mucous membranes, shock, bradyarrhythmias, and cardiac output by increasing strength of contraction.

Hazards

Do not give with epinephrine. May cause tremors, palpitation. Severe symptoms may include acute cardiac dilation, pulmonary edema. The effect of the drug may be blocked by giving propranolol, even when given after aerosolized Isuprel.

Metaproterenol Sulfate (Alupent)

Drug Type

Synthetic sympathetic agent

Drug Dose

20 mg tid or qid orally, 0.3 ml in 3 ml saline by nebulizer q4 – 6h; 0.65 mg/inhalation, no more than 12 inhalations/day

Remarks

A bronchodilator used to reverse bronchospasm associated with bronchitis, emphysema, and other pulmonary disease. Effects may last for 4 to 6 hours.

Hazards

Contraindicated with cardiac arrhythmias, tachycardia. Caution should be used when giving this drug to patients with hypertension, coronary artery disease, congestive heart failure, hyperthyroidism, or diabetes mellitus.

Normal Saline

Drug Type

Diluent

Drug Dose

1 to 3 ml of 0.9% solution

Remarks

Physiologic diluent for many aerosol preparations

Hazards

Some patients may have bronchospasms when inhaling normal saline.

Phenylephrine Hydrochloride (Neo-Synephrine)

Drug Type

Synthetic sympathetic agent

Drug Dose

10 mg q3–4h prn orally, 1 to 10 mg prn parenterally, 0.125% to 0.5% solution q3–4h prn topically

Remarks

Administered to produce vasoconstriction. Sometimes given with bronchodilators to enhance and prolong their action. Taken nasally as a decongestant. Directly affects α-adrenergic receptors. Effect seen within minutes after inhalation and lasts 3 to 4 hours.

Hazards

Lightheadedness, palpitation, tingling in extremities, and nervousness. With overdose, headache, hypertension, arrhythmias, convulsions, cerebral hemorrhage. Not to be given to patients with histories of cardiac arrhythmias, hypertension, or narrow-angle glaucoma.

Potassium Iodide (SSKI)

Drug Type

Expectorant

Drug Dose

0.3 to 0.6 ml (300–600 mg) PO tid or qid

Remarks

Used as an expectorant

Hazards

Not to be used in thyroid disturbances, tuberculosis, or in acute inflammatory conditions. This solution has an unpleasant taste. May be diluted in milk.

Propylene Glycol

Drug Type

Diluent

Drug Dose

2% to 10% 1 to 5 ml

Remarks

Used as a diluent or carrier with other mucokinetic agents. Sometimes used as an antiseptic on staphylococci, but is not effective on bacterial spores.

Hazards

Only if obtaining sputum samples; value may give false results because of antiseptic.

Pyridostigmine Bromide (Mestinon)

Drug Type

Cholinesterase inhibitor

Drug Dose

600 mg to 1.5 g in divided doses orally, 5 mg/ml injection

Remarks

Used for myasthenia gravis. The drug is a reversible cholinesterase inhibitor, with a long duration of action.

Hazards

Not to be used in patients with intestinal or urinary blockage, or if the patient is bradycardic. This drug is not to be used with depolarizing neuromuscular blocking agents. Use caution when giving this drug to bronchial asthma patients.

RESUSCITATION OR EMERGENCY DRUGS

Atropine

Drug Type

Parasympatholytic; *Atropa belladonna*

Drug Dose

IM, 0.1 mg/ml; IV bolus, 0.5 to 1.0 mg = 5 to 10 ml. Do not exceed 2 mg.

Remarks

Treatment of sinus bradycardia, to increase respiratory rate, relax smooth muscle tissue.

Hazards

Reduction of bronchial secretions, pupil dilation, dry mouth, tachycardia, and increase in blood pressure.

Bretylium Tosylate (Bretylol)

Drug Type

Sympathetic

Drug Dose

5 mg/kg, 350 to 500 mg as initial dose in 5% dextrose in water

Remarks

Treatment of ventricular tachycardia or ventricular fibrillation when first-line agents have failed.

Hazards

Hypotension in supine patients. May cause nausea, vomiting, bradycardia, increase in the number of premature ventricular contractions. When giving this drug you should monitor ECG.

Calcium Chloride

Drug Type

Essential electrolyte

Drug Dose

500 mg = 5 ml

Remarks

Increase myocardial tone and contractility in cardiac arrest. Increase in coarseness of fibrillatory waves in ventricular fibrillation.

Hazards

Tissue sloughing and necrosis caused by IV infiltrate. May precipitate bradycardia, arrhythmias, and arrest. Monitor ECG.

Dopamine (Intropin, Dobutrex)

Drug Type

Sympathetic

Drug Dose

Infusion, 1 to 10 μg/kg/minute

Remarks

Short-term treatment of cardiac decompensation due to depressed contractility (hypotension), which may be due to shock. This is a direct-acting inotropic agent that stimulates β receptors of the heart.

Hazards

Increase in heart rate, systolic blood pressure, nausea, headache, anginal pain, and tissue sloughing. Monitor ECG, blood pressure, and pulmonary wedge pressure.

Epinephrine (Adrenalin)

Drug Type

Natural sympathetic (animal glands)

Drug Dose

0.5 mg to 1.0 mg = 5 to 10 ml IV or intratracheal

Remarks

Initiates cardiac rhythm in cardiac standstill. Drug acts directly on both α- and β-adrenergic receptors.

Hazards

Epinephrine can interact with cyclopropane and other halogenated hydrocarbon anesthetics to cause cardiac arrhythmias. May cause ventricular dysrhythmias and reduce renal blood flow.

Isoproterenol (Isuprel)

Drug Type

Sympathetic stimulant

Drug Dose

Infusion, 2 to 20 μg/minute; 1 mg in 5% dextrose in water

Remarks

Increases cardiac output, enhances pacemaker and atrioventricular conduction during heart block (see under respiratory drugs).

Hazards

Severe symptoms are acute cardiac dilation and pulmonary edema.

Lidocaine (Xylocaine)

Drug Type

Cardiac depressant

Drug Dose

Infusion, 1 to 4 mg/minute. For breakthrough ventricular ectopy, additional 50-mg bolus every 5 minutes or total of 225 mg.

Remarks

Treatment of ventricular dysrhythmias by increasing electrical stimulation threshold of ventricles during diastole.

Hazards

Hypotension, disorientation, depressed reflexes, and circulatory collapse.

Methoxamine Hydrochloride

Drug Type

Synthetic sympathetic agent

Drug Dose

5 to 20 mg prn IM, IV

Remarks

Used to increase blood pressure. This drug is a strong vasopressor by causing constriction of peripheral blood vessels.

Hazards

Possible high blood pressure, weakness, chest pain, tremors, and respiratory distress.

Propranolol (Inderal)

Drug Type

Beta-adrenergic blocking agent

Drug Dose

1 to 3 mg IV given under ECG monitoring; not to exceed 1 mg/minute

Remarks

This drug is used for life-threatening arrhythmias or those occurring under anesthesia. Can be used for hypertension, angina pectoris, cardiac arrhythmias, hypertrophic subaortic stenosis, and prevention of migraines.

Hazards

Nausea, vomiting, mental depression, fever with sore throat, and hallucinations. Not to be used for patients with bronchial asthma, allergic rhinitis, sinus bradycardia, heart block, or congestive heart failure.

Sodium Bicarbonate

Drug Type

Alkaline

Drug Dose

1 mEq/kg or 75 ml initial dose (average-size adult)

Remarks

Decreases acidity; can be used as a mucolytic.

Hazards

Excessive amounts may cause alkalosis.

Sodium Nitroprusside

Drug Type

Vasodilator antihypertensive

Drug Dose

0.1 to 0.6 mg prn orally, 2.5 to 6.5 mg bid sublingually, 2% ointment topically.

Remarks

To treat hypertension crisis, control hypotension during anesthesia. Hypotensive effect caused by direct action on blood vessels, leading to peripheral vasodilation.

Hazards

Nausea, diaphoresis, headache, palpitations, and abdominal pain. Should monitor thiocyanate blood levels.

DRUGS USED IN CARDIAC ARREST

Table 8–1 details the drugs used in cardiac arrest.

AEROSOL ANTIVIRAL INHIBITOR
Virazole (Ribavirin)

Drug Type

Antiviral inhibitor

Drug Dose

20 mg/ml in 300 ml of sterile USP water, for a 12-hour period for aerosol therapy using only a SPAG-2 unit for delivery of this drug

Remarks

Ribavirin has antiviral inhibitory activity in vitro against respiratory syncytial virus, influenza virus, herpes simplex virus.

Hazards

Contraindicated in women or girls who are or may become

Table 8-1. DRUGS USED IN CARDIAC ARREST:
HOW SUPPLIED, USUAL DOSE (AVERAGE ADULT)

Drug	Concentration and Volume of Prefilled Syringe	Dose	Infusion Rate	Remarks
Atropine sulfate	0.1 mg/ml in 10-ml syringe	0.5 – 1.0 mg = 5 – 10 ml	. . .	Repeat at 5-minute intervals to achieve desired rate. Generally, do not exceed 2 mg
Bretylium tosylate	50 mg/ml in 10-ml ampule	5 mg/kg 350 – 500 mg as initial dose	500 mg in 5% dextrose in water (in 250 ml = 2 mg/ml; in 500 ml = 1 mg/ml) Infusion: 1 – 2 mg/minute	Infusion started after loading dose to control recurrent ventricular tachycardia or ventricular fibrillation
Calcium chloride 10%	500 mg/ml in 10-ml syringe	500 mg = 5 ml	. . .	May repeat dose every 10 minutes as needed

(*continued*)

259

Table 8–1. Continued

Drug	Concentration and Volume of Prefilled Syringe	Dose	Infusion Rate	Remarks
Dopamine	200 mg in 5-ml ampule	...	200 mg in 250 ml dextrose in water = 800 μg/ml Infusion: 2 – 10 μg/kg/minute	...
Epinephrine 1 : 10,000	0.1 mg/ml in 10-ml syringe	0.5 – 1.0 mg = 5 – 10 ml IV or intratracheal	1 mg in 5% dextrose in water (in 250 ml = 4 μg/ml; in 500 ml = 2 μg/ml) Infusion: 1 μg/minute for maintenance of blood pressure	Avoid intracardiac injection. Repeat dose every 5 minutes as needed in cardiac arrest
Isoproterenol	0.1 mg/ml in 5-ml ampule	...	1 mg in 5% dextrose in water (in 250 ml = 4 μg/ml; in 500 ml = 2 μg/ml) Infusion: 2 – 20 μg/minute. Titrate	Beware of premature ventricular contractions
Lidocaine	For IV bolus 1% (10 mg/ml) in 10 ml = 100 mg 2% (20 mg/ml) in 5 ml = 100 mg	1%: 75 mg = 7.50 ml 2%: 75 mg = 3.75 ml	2 g in 500 ml 5% dextrose in water (or 1 g in 250 ml) = 4 mg/ml Infusion: 1 – 4 mg/minute	For breakthrough ventricular ectopy: additional 50-mg bolus every 5 minutes to

	Preparation	Dosage	IV infusion	Comments
	For infusion after bolus: 4% (40 mg/ml) in 25 ml = 1 g			suppress, or total of 225 mg. Increase drip to 4 mg/minute
Procainamide	For IV bolus: 100 mg/ml in 10-ml ampule. For infusion after bolus: 500 mg/ml in 2-ml ampules	20 mg/minute until: a) Dysrhythmia suppressed b) Hypotension c) QRS widens by 50% d) Total 1 g administered	1 g in 250 ml 5% dextrose—4 mg/ml. Infusion: 1–4 mg/minute	Monitor ECG and blood pressure. Administer cautiously in patients with acute myocardial infarction
Sodium bicarbonate	1 mEq/ml in 50 ml = 50 mEq	1 mEq/kg or 75 ml initial dose (average-size adult) or preferably according to pH	. . .	Repeat according to pH. If not available, use ½ initial dose every 10 minutes

(From McIntyre, JD: Textbook of Advanced Cardiac Life Support. American Heart Association, Dallas, 1983, with permission.)

pregnant during exposure to this drug. *Please read the warning label of this or any other drug before using.*

BIBLIOGRAPHY

The works listed below are also suggested readings that will give the reader more information concerning the chapter content.

Baker, CE: Physician's Desk Reference. Medical Economics, Oradell, NJ, 1987.

Bergersen, BS: Pharmacology in Nursing. CV Mosby, St. Louis, 1973.

McIntyre, JD: Textbook of Advanced Cardiac Life Support. American Heart Association, Dallas, 1983.

Mathewson, MK: Pharmacotherapeutics. FA Davis, Philadelphia, 1986.

Patterson, R: Current Drug Handbook. WB Saunders, Philadelphia, 1986.

NOTES

NOTES

9 **Medical Terminology***

Basic Word Structure
Respiratory Terms

This chapter provides a review of respiratory terminology as well as of the basic word structure of medical terms.

BASIC WORD STRUCTURE

Most medical words can be broken down into four word parts.

The root word—contains the meaning of the word.

The suffix—attached to the end of the root word, which when added will alter the root word.

The prefix—is added to the front of the root word, which can change the meaning of the root word or make a new word.

The combining form—is the root word with a combining vowel, which is usually the letter o.

An example is the following:

Electro/cardi/o/gram

cardi-   root word

electro- prefix

gram-   suffix

cardi/o- combining vowel and form

---

*The author and publisher have exerted every effort to ensure that the respiratory terminology in this text is in accord with current recommendations and practice at the time of publication. However, in view of ongoing research and advances in the field of respiratory care, the reader should refer to listings under the American College of Chest Physicians for any questionable term.

By taking the medical term and breaking it down into the root word, suffix, prefix, and the combining form you can start to define most terms.

When defining medical terms, usually the suffix is defined first, then the rest of the word.

RESPIRATORY TERMS

Table 9–1 defines terms used by the respiratory care practitioner as they apply to the field of respiratory care.

Table 9–1. RESPIRATORY TERMS

Terms	Definitions
acidosis	An abnormal increase in hydrogen ion concentration in the body, which will decrease the pH below 7.35. It may be caused by an increased carbon dioxide level or a decreased amount of base or even by a combination of both an increased carbon dioxide and a decreasing base.
aerosol	Liquid particles suspended in a gas.
airway pressure	Indicates the amount of pressure placed or applied to the upper airways during inspiration or expiration, usually measured with a manometer.

(continued)

Table 9-1 — *Continued*

Terms	Definitions
alkalosis	An abnormal decrease in hydrogen ion concentration in the body, which will increase the pH above 7.45. It may be caused by a decreased carbon dioxide level or an increased amount of base, or by a combination of both a decreased carbon dioxide level and an increasing base.
alveolar-arterial gradient $(P_{(A}-a)_{O_2})$	The difference in partial pressure of oxygen in alveolar gas and that of arterial blood.
alveolar ventilation	Tidal volume minus dead space, or the volume of gas in the alveoli that can be available for perfusion.
apnea	Complete absence of ventilation.
apnea alarm	Any type of system that senses the absence of ventilation. These alarms may be found on ventilators, in sleep labs, and in home care.
arterial-venous oxygen difference $((Ca-C\bar{v})_{O_2})$	Difference in oxygen content between arterial and mixed venous (pulmonary artery) blood.

(continued)

Table 9–1 — *Continued*

Terms	Definitions
arterial blood gas analysis (ABG)	Used to determine pH, carbon dioxide, oxygen, oxygen saturation, bicarbonate, and base excess levels.
assist	Control found on some ventilators that when used will respond only during the patient's inspiratory effort.
assist/control	A ventilator mode used as an assist with a controlled back-up rate; if the patient fails to initiate an assist breath, the ventilator will deliver one at a predetermined control rate.
bradypnea	A very slow rate of breathing.
cardiac output (CO)	The amount of blood the heart pumps out of the ventricles per minute. The normal adult value is about 5 L/minute.
central venous pressure (CVP)	Blood pressure measurement reflective of right heart filling pressure. Normal adult parameter for CVP is 5 to 15 cmH$_2$O.
compliance (normal is 100 ml/cmH$_2$O) $$C = \frac{\text{change in volume}}{\text{change in pressure}}$$	Forces resisting the expansion of the lung, or the "distensibility of the lung." *(continued)*

Table 9–1 — *Continued*

Terms	Definitions
dynamic (C_D or C_{Dyn})	Compliance of the lung measured during flow or movement of a gas.
static (C_s or C_{stat})	Compliance of the lung and thorax, measured when there is no gas movement.
tubing and machine	Compliance of the ventilator and ventilator tubing.
continuous positive airway pressure (CPAP)	Constant positive pressure delivered to the patient throughout the ventilatory cycle. Note that the patient must have a spontaneous breathing rate before CPAP can be used.
control ventilation	Any type of ventilation that allows the patient no control over the rate or volume. Each breath is dictated by the ventilator for each breath.
dead space (V_D or ds)	Volume of gas that does not participate in gas exchange, both mechanical and patient volumes.
elastance, elasticity ($\frac{1}{C}$)	The ability of a substance to return to its original shape after being stretched, the reciprocal of compliance.
exudate	Discharge of fluid from cells or blood vessels.

(continued)

Table 9–1 — *Continued*

Terms	Definitions
forced vital capacity (FVC)	Volume of gas measured at the end of a forced maximum exhalation, after a maximum inspiration.
frequency (f)	Ventilatory or respiratory rate.
humidifier	Any device that can add water to a gas.
hypercarbia	Carbon dioxide level above normal range; for arterial blood, amounts above 45 mmHg.
hyperventilation	Faster than normal ventilatory rate, or an increase in minute volume by increasing the rate and/or depth of breathing, or ventilation in excess of metabolic demands.
hypocarbia	Carbon dioxide level below normal range; in arterial blood this is usually a Pa_{CO_2} of below 35 mmHg at sea level.
inflation hold	A pause at the end of inspiration and before the start of exhalation.
I : E ratio	The ratio of time devoted to inspiration (I) and expiratory (E) time

(*continued*)

Table 9–1 — *Continued*

Terms	Definitions
	expressed as a proportion equaling the total cycle time of one breath.
inspiratory flow rate	The volume of gas delivered per unit of time, usually noted in liters per minute or liters per second.
inspiratory time	The time period from the start to the end of the inspiratory cycle.
intermittent mandatory ventilation (IMV)	Spontaneous breathing aided by periods of controlled breaths from a ventilator.
maximum inspiratory pressure (MIP)	Highest pressure reached during inspiration as shown on a pressure manometer.
mucopurulent	Sputum that contains a combination of mucus and pus.
mucus	Viscous, slippery secretions of the mucous membranes and glands, which contain mucin, white blood cells, water, inorganic salts, and exfoliated cells.
orthopnea	Difficulty in breathing while lying down.
oxygen content (normal 16–20 ml/100 ml)	Amount of oxygen carried in the blood.

(*continued*)

Table 9-1 — *Continued*

Terms	Definitions
oxygen saturation (normal >95%)	The fraction of a total hemoglobin in the form of HbO_2 at a defined P_{O_2}.
pop-off valves	Usually adjustable safety systems allowing for excess gas flow or pressure to escape the system.
positive end-expiratory pressure (PEEP)	Positive pressure left in the airway even after exhalation. Usually used to imply use with mechanical ventilation.
purulent (sputum)	A pale yellow to yellow-green sputum containing pus.
retraction (breathing)	Visible sinking in of the soft tissue at the intercostal space margins during an inspiratory effort.
shunt	The amount of blood that flows through circulation without undergoing gas exchange.
static pressure	No gas flow through a system. The pressure is equal to the elastic recoil of that system, usually referring to the lung's elastic recoil.
tachypnea	A ventilatory rate above normal, sometimes thought of as a rate

(continued)

Table 9–1 — *Continued*

Terms	Definitions
	greater than 20 breaths per minute in an adult.
tidal volume (Vt)	The amount of gas that is inhaled or exhaled during a normal breath.
triggering (or assisting)	Negative inspiratory pressure generated by the patient to initiate a breath in an assist mode of ventilation.
ventilator	Any device that can mechanically provide a volume or pressure to ventilate a patient's lungs.
viscid	Sticky or glutinous sputum or fluids.

BIBLIOGRAPHY

The works listed below are also suggested readings that will give the reader more information concerning the chapter content.

Abels, MN: Mosby's Manual of Critical Care. St. Louis, CV Mosby, 1979.

Chabner, DE: The Language of Medicine, ed 3. Philadelphia, WB Saunders, 1985.

Gylys, B and Wedding, MH: Medical Terminology: A Systems Approach, ed 2. FA Davis, Philadelphia, 1988.

Thomas, CL (ed): Taber's Cyclopedic Medical Dictionary, ed 15. FA Davis, Philadelphia, 1985.

NOTES

Appendices

APPENDIX 1. UNITS OF MEASUREMENT

Scientific Notation

Sometimes it is necessary to use very large and very small numbers. These can best be indicated and handled in calculations by use of exponents. Use of scientific notation, which is to say by use of exponents. Use of scientific notation requires writing the number so that it is the result of multiplying some whole number power of 10 by a number between 1 and 10. Examples are:

$$1234 = 1.234 \times 10^3 \qquad\qquad 0.01234 = 1.234 \times \frac{1}{100} = 1.234 \times 10^{-2}$$

$$0.001234 = 1.234 \times \frac{1}{1000} = 1.234 \times 10^{-3}$$

To convert a number to its equivalent in scientific notation:

Place the decimal point to the right of the first non-zero digit. This will now be a number between 1 and 9.

Multiply this number by a power of 10, the exponent of which is equal to the number of places the decimal point was moved. The exponent is positive if the decimal point was moved to the left, and negative if it was moved to the right. For example:

$$\frac{1,234,000.0 \times 0.000072}{6000.0} = \frac{1.234 \times 10^6 \times 7.2 \times 10^{-5}}{6.0 \times 10^3}$$

Now, by simply adding or subtracting the exponents of ten, and remembering that moving an exponent from the denominator of the fraction to the numerator changes its sign,

$$= \frac{1.234 \times 10^6 \times 10^{-5} \times 10^{-3} \times 7.2}{6} = \frac{1.234 \times 10^{-2} \times 7.2}{6}$$

Now, dividing by 6,

$$= 1.234 \times 10^{-2} \times 1.2 = 1.4808 \times 10^{-2} = \frac{1.4808}{100} = 0.014808$$

The last operation changed 1.4808×10^{-2} into the final value, 0.014808, which is not expressed in scientific notation.

Metric System

Weights

Scale	Table		Grams		Grains
Kilo	1 Kilogram	=	1000.0	=	15,432.35
Hecto	1 Hectogram	=	100.0	=	1,543.23
Deca	1 Decagram	=	10.0	=	154.323
Unit	1 Gram	=	1.0	=	15.432
Deci	1 Decigram	=	0.1	=	1.5432
Centi	1 Centigram	=	0.01	=	0.15432
Milli	1 Milligram	=	0.001	=	0.01543
Micro	1 Microgram	=	10^{-6}	=	15.432×10^{-6}
Nano	1 Nanogram	=	10^{-9}	=	15.432×10^{-9}
Pico	1 Picogram	=	10^{-12}	=	15.432×10^{-12}
Femto	1 Femtogram	=	10^{-15}	=	15.432×10^{-15}
Atto	1 Attogram	=	10^{-18}	=	15.432×10^{-18}

Arabic numbers are used with weights and measures, as 10 gm., or 3 ml., etc. Portions of weights and measures are usually expressed decimally. 10^{-1} indicates 0.1; $10^{-6} = 0.000001$; etc. SEE: *Scientific Notation* in *Appendix*.

55555555555

SI Units (Système international d'Units) or International System of Units

This system includes two types of units important in clinical medicine. The *base units* are shown in the first table, derived units in the second table, and derived units with special names in the third table.

SI Base Units

Quantity	Name	Symbol
Length	meter	m
Mass	kilogram	kg
Time	second	s
Electric current	ampere	A
Temperature	kelvin	K
Luminous intensity	candela	cd
Amount of a substance	mole	mol

Some SI Derived Units

Quantity	Name of Derived Unit	Symbol
Area	square meter	m^2
Volume	cubic meter	m^3
Speed, velocity	meter per second	m/s
Acceleration	meter per second squared	m/s^2
Density	kilogram per cubic meter	kg/m^3
Concentration of a substance	mole per cubic meter	mol/m^3
Specific volume	cubic meter per kilogram	m^3/kg
Luminescence	candela per square meter	cd/m^2

SI Derived Names With Special Names

Quantity	Name	Symbol	Expressed in Terms of Other Units
Frequency	hertz	Hz	S^{-1}
Force	newton	N	$kg \cdot m \cdot s^{-2}$ or $kg \cdot m/s^2$
Pressure	pascal	Pa	$N \cdot m^{-2}$ or N/m^2
Energy, work, amount of heat	joule	j	$N \cdot m$
Power	watt	W	$j \cdot s$ or j/s
Quantity of electricity	coulomb	C	$A \cdot s$
Electromotive force	volt	V	W/A
Capacitance	farad	F	C/V
Electrical resistance	ohm	Ω	V/a
Conductance	siemens	S	A/V
Inductance	henry	H	$W\phi/A$
Illuminance	lux	lx	ln/m^2
Absorbed (radiation) dose	gray	Gy	J/kg

Prefixes and Multiples Used in SI

Prefix	Symbol	Power	Multiple or Portion of a Multiple
tera	T	10^{12}	1,000,000,000,000
giga	G	10^9	1,000,000,000
mega	M	10^6	1,000,000
kilo	k	10^3	1,000
hecto	h	10^2	100
deca	da	10^1	10
unity			1
deci	d	10^{-1}	0.1
centi	c	10^{-2}	0.01
milli	m	10^{-3}	0.001
micro	μ	10^{-6}	0.000001
nano	n	10^{-9}	0.000000001
pico	p	10^{-12}	0.000000000001
femto	f	10^{-15}	0.000000000000001
atto	a	10^{-18}	0.000000000000000001

Tables of Data

Arabic numerals are used with weights and measures, as 10 gm., or 3 ml., etc. Portions of weights and measures are usually expressed decimally. For practical purposes, 1 cc. (cubic centimeter) is equivalent to 1 ml. (milliliter) and 1 drop (gtt) of water is equivalent to a minim (m).

Units of Length

Millimeters	Centimeters	Inches	Feet	Yards	Meters
1 mm. = 1.0	0.1	0.03937	0.00328	0.0011	0.001
1 cm. = 10.0	1.0	0.3937	0.03281	0.0109	0.01
1 in. = 25.4	2.54	1.0	0.0833	0.0278	0.0254
1 ft. = 304.8	30.48	12.0	1.0	0.333	0.3048
1 yd. = 914.40	91.44	36.0	3.0	1.0	0.9144
1 m. = 1000.0	100.0	39.37	3.2808	1.0936	1.0

$1 \mu = 1$ **mu** $= 1$ **micrometer** $= 0.001$ millimeter. 1 mm. $= 1000 \mu$.
1 km. = 1 kilometer = 1000 meters = 0.6215 mile.
1 mile = 5280 feet = 1.609 kilometers.

Units of Volume (fluid or liquid)

Milliliters		U.S. Fluid Drams	Cubic Inches	U.S. Fluid Ounces	U.S. Fluid Quarts	Liters
1 ml.	= 1.0	0.2705	0.061	0.03381	0.00106	0.001
1 fl. ʒ	= 3.697	1.0	0.226	0.125	0.00391	0.00369
1 cu. in.	= 16.3866	4.4329	1.0	0.5541	0.0173	0.01639
1 fl. ʒ	= 29.573	8.0	1.8047	1.0	0.03125	0.02957
1 qt.	= 946.332	256.0	57.75	32.0	1.0	0.9463
1 L.	= 1000.0	270.52	61.025	33.815	1.0567	1.0

1 gallon = 4 quarts = 8 pints = 3.785 liters.
1 pint = 473.16 ml.

Units of Weight

Grains		Grams	Apothecaries' Ounces	Avoirdupois Pounds	Kilograms
1 gr.	= 1.0	0.0648	0.00208	0.0001429	0.000065
1 gm.	= 15.432	1.0	0.03215	0.002205	0.001
1 ʒ	= 480.0	31.1	1.0	0.06855	0.0311
1 lb.	= 7000.0	453.5924	14.583	1.0	0.45354
1 kg.	= 15432.358	1000.0	32.15	2.2046	1.0

1 γ = 1 gamma = 1 microgram = 0.001 milligram; 1000 γ = 1 mg.
1 mg. = 1 milligram = 0.001 gm.; 1000 mg. = 1 gm.
1 grain = 64.8 mg.; 1 mg. = 0.0154 grain.
NOTE: 1 microgram may also be expressed as 1 μg.

Weights* and Measures

Apothecaries' Weight

20 grains = 1 scruple
8 drams = 1 ounce

3 scruples = 1 dram
12 ounces = 1 pound

Avoirdupois Weight

27.343 grains = 1 dram
16 ounces = 1 pound
2000 pounds = 1 short ton
1 oz. troy = 480 grains
1 lb. troy = 5760 grains

16 drams = 1 ounce
100 pounds = 1 hundredweight
2240 pounds = 1 long ton
1 oz. avoirdupois = 437.5 grains
1 lb. avoirdupois = 7000 grains

Circular Measure

60 seconds = 1 minute
90 degrees = 1 quadrant

60 minutes = 1 degree
4 quadrants = 360 degrees = circle

Cubic Measure

1728 cubic inches = 1 cubic foot
2150.42 cubic inches = 1 standard bushel
1 cubic foot = about four-fifths of a bushel

27 cubic feet = 1 cubic yard
268.8 cubic inches = 1 dry (U.S.) gallon
128 cubic feet = 1 cord (wood)

Dry Measure

2 pints = 1 quart   8 quarts = 1 peck   4 pecks = 1 bushel

Liquid Measure

16 ounces = 1 pint
1000 milliliters = 1 liter
4 gills = 1 pint

4 quarts = 1 gallon
31.5 gallons = 1 barrel (U.S.)
2 pints = 1 quart

2 barrels = 1 hogshead (U.S.)
1 quart = 0.946 liters

Barrels and hogsheads vary in size. A U.S. gallon is equal to 0.8327 British gallon; therefore a British
gallon is equal to 1.201 U.S. gallons.
1 liter is equal to 1.0567 quarts.

Linear Measure

1 inch = 2.54 centimeters
12 inches = 1 foot
1 statute mile = 5280 feet

40 rods = 1 furlong
3 feet = 1 yard
3 statute miles = 1 statute league

8 furlongs = 1 statute mile
5.5 yards = 1 rod

Troy Weight

24 grains = 1 pennyweight   20 pennyweights = 1 ounce   12 ounces = 1 pound
Used for weighing gold, silver, and jewels.

*For abbreviations and symbols of these weights, see *Symbols* in *Appendix*.

Household Measures* and Weights

Approximate Equivalents: 60 gtt. = 1 teaspoonful = 5 ml.
= 60 minims = 60 grains = 1 dram = ⅛ ounce

1 teaspoon = ⅛ fl. oz.; 1 dram
3 teaspoons = 1 tablespoon
1 tablespoon = ½ fl. oz.; 4 drams

16 tablespoons (liquid) = 1 cup
12 tablespoons (dry) = 1 cup
1 cup = 8 fl. oz.

1 tumbler or glass = 8 fl. oz.; ½ pint

*Household measures are not precise. For instance, household tsp. will hold from 3 to 5 ml. of liquid
substances. Therefore, do not substitute household equivalents for medication prescribed by the
physician.

Conversion Rules

To convert units of one system into the other, multiply the number of units in column I by the equivalent factor opposite that unit in column II.

Weight

I		II
1 milligram	=	0.015432 grain
1 gram	=	15.432 grains
1 gram	=	0.25720 apothecaries' dram
1 gram	=	0.03527 avoirdupois ounce
1 gram	=	0.03215 apothecaries' or troy ounce
1 kilogram	=	35.274 avoirdupois ounces
1 kilogram	=	32.151 apothecaries' or troy ounces
1 kilogram	=	2.2046 avoirdupois pounds
1 grain	=	64.7989 milligrams
1 grain	=	0.0648 gram
1 apothecaries' dram	=	3.8879 gram
1 avoirdupois ounce	=	28.3495 grams
1 apothecaries' or troy ounce	=	31.1035 grams
1 avoirdupois pound	=	453.5924 grams

Volume (air or gas)

I		II
1 cubic centimeter	=	0.06102 cubic inch
1 cubic meter	=	35.314 cubic feet
1 cubic meter	=	1.3079 cubic yard
1 cubic inch	=	16.3872 cubic centimeters
1 cubic foot	=	0.02832 cubic meter

Capacity (fluid or liquid)

I		II
1 milliliter	=	16.23 minims
1 milliliter	=	0.2705 fluid dram
1 milliliter	=	0.0338 fluid ounce
1 liter	=	33.8148 fluid ounces
1 liter	=	2.1134 pints
1 liter	=	1.0567 quart
1 liter	=	0.2642 gallon
1 fluid dram	=	3.697 milliliters
1 fluid ounce	=	29.573 milliliters
1 pint	=	473.166 milliliters
1 quart	=	946.332 milliliters
1 gallon	=	3.785 liters

To Convert Centigrade or Celsius Degrees to Fahrenheit Degrees*

Multiply the number of Centigrade degrees by $\frac{9}{5}$ and add 32 to the result.

Example: $55° \text{ C.} \times \frac{9}{5} = 99 + 32 = 131° \text{ F.}$

To convert Fahrenheit degrees to Centigrade degrees: Subtract 32 from the number of Fahrenheit degrees and multiply the difference by $\frac{5}{9}$.

Example: $243° \text{ F.} - 32 = 211 \times \frac{5}{9} = 117.2° \text{ C.}$

*SEE: *thermometry* for table.

Miscellaneous Conversion Factors

Pressure

to obtain	multiply	by
lb./sq. in.	atmospheres	14.696
lb./sq. in.	in. of water	0.03609
lb./sq. in.	ft. of water	0.4335
lb./sq. in.	in. of mercury	0.4912
lb./sq. in.	kg./sq. meter	0.00142
lb./sq. in.	kg./sq. cm.	14.22
lb./sq. in.	cm. of mercury	0.1934
lb./sq. ft.	atmospheres	2116.8
lb./sq. ft.	in. of water	5.204
lb./sq. ft.	ft. of water	62.48
lb./sq. ft.	in. of mercury	70.727
lb./sq. ft.	cm. of mercury	27.845
lb./sq. ft.	kg./sq. meter	0.20482
lb./cu. ft.	gm./ml.	0.03613
lb./cu. ft.	lb./cu. in.	1728.0
lb./cu. ft.	gm./ml.	62.428
lb./U.S. gal.	gm./l.	8.345
in. of water	in. of mercury	13.60
in. of water	cm. of mercury	5.3543
ft. of water	atmospheres	33.95
ft. of water	lb./sq. in.	2.307
ft. of water	kg./sq. meter	0.00328
ft. of water	in. of mercury	1.133
ft. of water	cm. of mercury	0.4461
atmospheres	ft. of water	0.02947
atmospheres	in. of mercury	0.03342
atmospheres	kg./sq. cm.	0.9678
bars	atmospheres	1.0133
in. of mercury	atmospheres	29.921
in. of mercury	lb./sq. in.	2.036
mm. of mercury	atmospheres	760.0
gm./ml.	lb./cu. in.	27.68
gm./sq. cm.	kg./sq. meter	0.1
kg./sq. meter	lb./sq. in.	703.1
kg./sq. meter	in. of water	25.40
kg./sq. meter	in. of mercury	345.32
kg./sq. meter	cm. of mercury	135.95
kg./sq. meter	atmospheres	10332.0
kg./sq. cm.	atmospheres	1.0332

Flow Rate

To obtain	multiply	by
cu. ft./hr.	cc./min.	0.00212
cu. ft./hr.	L./min.	2.12
L./min.	cu. ft./hr.	0.472

Parts Per Million

Conversion of parts per million (ppm) to percent: 1 ppm = 0.0001%, 10 ppm = 0.001%, 100 ppm = 0.01%, 1000 ppm = 0.1%, 10,000 ppm = 1%, etc.

Miscellaneous Units of Measurement

Units of Time

1 millisecond = one thousandth (0.001) of a second
1 second = $\frac{1}{60}$ of a minute

1 minute = $\frac{1}{60}$ of an hour
1 hour = $\frac{1}{24}$ of a day

Units of Temperature

Given a temperature on the Fahrenheit scale; to convert it to Centigrade, subtract 32 and multiply by $\frac{5}{9}$. Given a temperature on the Centigrade scale; to convert it to Fahrenheit, multiply by $\frac{9}{5}$ and add 32. Celsius degrees are equivalent to Centigrade degrees.

Units of Energy

1 gram/centimeter = 980.665 dynes/centimeter
1 foot-pound = 13,558,200 ergs = 13,825.5 gram-centimeters
1 Joule = 0.2386 Calorie (kilocalorie)
1 Calorie = 4.26649×10^7 gram-centimeters = 3085.96 foot-pounds
1 Calorie (kilocalorie) = 1000 calories = 4184 Joules
A large Calorie, or kilocalorie, is always written with a capital C.

pH Table

The pH scale is simply a series of numbers stating where a given solution would stand in a series of solutions arranged according to acidity or alkalinity. At one extreme (i.e., high pH) lies an alkaline solution made by dissolving 4 gm. of sodium hydroxide in water to make a liter of solution; at the other is a solution containing 3.65 gm. of hydrogen chloride per liter. Halfway between lies purified water, which is neutral. All other solutions can be arranged on this scale, and their acidity or alkalinity can be stated by giving the numbers that indicate their relative positions.

Tenth-normal HCl	1.00	Litmus is red in
Gastric juice	*1.4	this acid range.
Urine	*6.0	
Water	7.00	Neutral
Blood	7.35–7.45	
Bile	*7.5	Litmus is blue in
Pancreatic juice	8.5	this alkaline range.
Tenth-normal NaOH	13.00	

If one is told that the pH of a certain solution is 5.3, one knows at once that it falls between gastric juice and urine on the above scale, is moderately acid, and will turn litmus red.

* These body fluids vary rather widely in pH; typical figures have been used for simplicity. Urine samples obtained from healthy individuals may have pH's anywhere between 4.7 and 8.0.

Preparation of Percentage Solutions

When the metric system is used, the preparation of percentage solutions is simple: a 1% solution contains 1 gm. in 100 ml.; a 0.1% solution contains 0.1 gm. (or 100 milligrams) per 100 ml.

When the apothecaries' system is used the following are helpful: 4.55 grains to the ounce, or 2.5 drams to 32 ounces; or 3.25 drams to 40 ounces, all make a 1% solution.

To Prepare a Dilute Solution From One Which Is Stronger:

For example, to make 80% alcohol from 95%: Dilute 80 ml. of the 95% alcohol to 95 ml. with distilled water.

Rule: Dilute a volume equal to the percent desired to a volume equal to the percent used.
SEE: *dosage.*

Percentage Solution Tables

Weight-in-volume solutions are prescribed by the USP to be used in compounding prescriptions whenever gases or solids are dissolved in liquids, since most physicians have in mind a certain weight of substance in a definite volume of solution. Such solutions are defined by the USP as "the number of grams of an active constituent in 100 milliliters of solution" regardless of whether water or some other liquid is the vehicle.

For such weight-in-volume solutions, the following tables will afford a ready means of ascertaining the quantities (by weight) of substance required to prepare varying volumes of definite w/v percentage strength. The calculations are based on 1 fl. oz. (480 minims) of water = 455 grains (round number) in the Apothecaries table and 100 ml. of water = 100 gm. in the Metric table.

For example, if 8 fluid ounces of a 0.5% solution of salt in water (% weight in volume) is needed, add 18.2 grains of salt to 8 fluid ounces of water. In the metric system, if 500 ml. of a 0.5% solution of salt in water (% weight in volume) is required, add 2.5 grams of salt to 500 ml. of water.

APOTHECARIES

	Grains of substance required per given volume of solution											
Strength of solution (% w/v)	¼ fl oz	½ fl oz	1 fl oz	2 fl oz	3 fl oz	4 fl oz	6 fl oz	8 fl oz	10 fl oz	12 fl oz	16 fl oz
0.01	0.0114	0.023	0.046	0.091	0.137	0.182	0.273	0.364	0.455	0.546	0.728
0.02	0.023	0.046	0.091	0.182	0.273	0.364	0.546	0.728	0.910	1.092	1.456
0.04	0.046	0.091	0.182	0.364	0.546	0.728	1.092	1.456	1.820	2.184	2.912
0.05	0.057	0.114	0.2275	0.455	0.683	0.910	1.365	1.820	2.275	2.730	3.640
0.1	0.114	0.228	0.455	0.910	1.365	1.820	2.730	3.640	4.55	5.46	7.28
0.2	0.2275	0.455	0.910	1.820	2.730	3.640	5.460	7.28	9.10	10.92	14.56
0.25	0.284	0.569	1.138	2.275	3.413	4.55	6.83	9.10	11.38	13.65	18.20
0.5	0.569	1.138	2.275	4.55	6.83	9.10	13.65	18.20	22.75	27.3	36.4
1	1.138	2.275	4.55	9.10	13.65	18.2	27.3	36.4	45.5	54.6	72.8
2	2.275	4.55	9.10	18.20	27.30	36.4	54.6	72.8	91.0	109.2	145.6
3	3.413	6.83	13.65	27.30	40.95	54.6	81.9	109.2	136.5	163.8	218.4
4	4.55	9.10	18.20	36.40	54.60	72.8	109.2	145.6	182.0	218.4	291.2
5	5.69	11.37	22.75	45.50	68.25	91.0	136.5	182.0	227.5	273	364
10	11.38	22.75	45.50	91.0	136.50	182	273	364	455	546	728
15	17.06	34.13	68.25	136.5	204.75	273	409.5	546	682.5	819	1092
20	22.75	45.50	91.0	182	273	364	546	728	910	1092	1456
25	28.44	56.90	113.75	227.5	341.25	455	682.5	910	1137.5	1365	1820
30	34.13	68.25	136.5	273	409.5	546	819	1092	1365	1638	2184
40	45.5	91.0	182	364	546	728	1092	1456	1820	2184	2912

METRIC

Strength of solution (% w/v)	Grams of substance required per given volume of solution											
	10 ml	15 ml	25 ml	30 ml	60 ml	90 ml	100 ml	120 ml	150 ml	200 ml	500 ml	1000 ml
0.01	0.001	0.0015	0.0025	0.003	0.006	0.009	0.01	0.012	0.015	0.02	0.05	0.1
0.02	0.002	0.003	0.005	0.006	0.012	0.018	0.02	0.024	0.03	0.04	0.1	0.2
0.05	0.005	0.008	0.013	0.015	0.03	0.045	0.05	0.06	0.075	0.1	0.25	0.5
0.1	0.01	0.015	0.025	0.03	0.06	0.09	0.1	0.12	0.15	0.2	0.5	1.0
0.2	0.02	0.03	0.05	0.06	0.12	0.18	0.2	0.24	0.30	0.4	1.0	2.0
0.25	0.025	0.038	0.063	0.075	0.15	0.225	0.25	0.3	0.375	0.5	1.25	2.5
0.5	0.05	0.075	0.125	0.15	0.3	0.45	0.5	0.6	0.75	1.0	2.5	5.0
1	0.1	0.15	0.25	0.3	0.6	0.9	1.0	1.2	1.5	2.0	5.0	10.0
1.5	0.15	0.225	0.375	0.45	0.9	1.35	1.5	1.8	2.25	3.0	7.5	15.0
2	0.2	0.3	0.5	0.6	1.2	1.8	2.0	2.4	3.0	4.0	10.0	20.0
3	0.3	0.45	0.75	0.9	1.8	2.7	3.0	3.6	4.5	6.0	15.0	30.0
4	0.4	0.6	1.0	1.2	2.4	3.6	4.0	4.8	6.0	8.0	20.0	40.0
5	0.5	0.75	1.25	1.5	3.0	4.5	5.0	6.0	7.5	10.0	25.0	50.0
10	1.0	1.5	2.5	3.0	6.0	9.0	10.0	12.0	15.0	20.0	50.0	100.0
15	1.5	2.25	3.75	4.5	9.0	13.5	15.0	18.0	22.5	30.0	75.0	150.0
20	2.0	3.0	5.0	6.0	12.0	18.0	20.0	24.0	30.0	40.0	100.0	200.0
25	2.5	3.75	6.25	7.5	15.0	22.5	25.0	30.0	37.5	50.0	125.0	250.0
40	4.0	6.0	10.0	12.0	24.0	36.0	40.0	48.0	60.0	80.0	200.0	400.0

From *Merck Index*, ed. 10, Merck & Co., Rahway, NJ, with permission.

APPENDIX 2. THE INTERPRETER

Basic Medical Diagnosis and Treatment

English, Spanish, Italian, French, German

Table of Contents

Introduction

When attempting to communicate with a person whose language is foreign to you it is important to establish that while you may be able to say a few words in his language you will not be able to understand the patient's replies. The patient may need to use signs in replying. The following paragraphs are given for your convenience in explaining your language difficulty to the patient.

English

Hello. I want to help you. I do not speak (English) but will use this book to ask you some questions. I will not be able to understand your spoken answers. Please respond by shaking your head or raising one finger to indicate "no"; nod your head or raise two fingers to indicate "yes."

Spanish

(Translation)

Saludos. Quiero ayudarlo. Yo no hablo español, pero voy a usar este libro para hacerle algunas preguntas. No voy a poder entender sus respuestas; por eso haga el favor de contestar, negando con la cabeza o levantando un dedo para indicar "no" y afirmando con la cabeza o levantando dos dedos para indicar "sí."

(Phonetic)

Sah-loo'dohs. Ki-air'oh ah-joo-dar'loh. Joh noh ah'bloh es'panyohl, pair'oh voy ah oo-sawr' es'tay lee'broh pahr'ah ah-sair'lay ahl-goo'nahs pray-goon'tahs. Noh voy ah poh-dair' en-ten-dair' soos res-poo-es'rahs; pore es-soh ah'gah el fah-vohr' day kohn-tes-tahr', nay-gahn'doh kohn lah kah-bay'thah oh lay-vahn-tahn'doh oon day'doh pahr'ah een-dee-kahr' noh ee ah-feer-mahn'doh kohn lah kah-bay'thah oh lay-vahn-tahn'doh days'dohs pahr'a een-dee-kahr' see.

Italian

(Translation)

Buon giorno. La voglio aiutare. Io non parlo italiano, ma userò questo libro per farle qualche domanda. Non potrò comprendere le Sue domande. Per favore risponda con un cenno di testa. Alzi un dito per indicare 'no'; muova la Sua testa su e giu o alzi due dita per indicare 'si.'

(Phonetic)

Bwon jih-or'noh. Lah vol'yoh ah-yoo-tar'day. Ee'oh nohn par'loh ee-towl-ee-ah'noh mah oo-say'roh kwes'toh lee'broh pehr fahr'lay kwall'kay doh-mahn'dah. Non poh'throh kohm-prehn'deh-ray lay soo'ee doh-mahn'day. Pehr fah-vohr'ay ray-spohn'dah kohn oon chay'noh dee tes'tah. Ahlt'zih oon dee'toh pehr in-dee-kar'ay noh; moo-eh'vah lah soo'ah tes'tah soo eh joo oh ahlt'zih doo'ay dee'tay pehr in-dee-kar'ay see.

French

(Translation)

Bonjour. Je veux bien vous aider. Je ne parle pas français mais tout en me servant de ce livre je vais vous poser des questions. Je ne comprendrai pas ce que vous dites en français. Je vous en prie, pour répondre: pour indiquer "non", secouez la tête ou levez un seul doigt; pour indiquer "oui", faites un signe de tête ou levez deux doigts.

(Phonetic)

Bon-zhoor'. Zheh voo bih-ehn' voo ay-day'. Zheh neh parl pah frahn-say' may too ahn meh sehr-vahn' d' seh lee'vrah zheh vay voo poh-say' day kehs-tih-on'. Zheh neh kahm-prahn'dry pah seh keh voo deet ahn frahn-say'. Zheh voo ahn pree, por ray-pahn'drah; por ahn-dee-kay nohn, seh-kway' lah teht oo leh-vay' oon sool dwoit; por ahn-dee-kay wee', fayt oon seen deh teht oo leh-vay' duh dwoit.

German

(Translation)

Hallo! Ich mochte Ihnen helfen. Ich spreche kein Deutsch, aber ich werde dieses Buch benützten um Sie einiges zu fragen. Ich werde Ihre Antworten nicht verstehen. Deshalb antworten Sie mir indem Sie Ihren Kopf schütteln oder heben Sie Ihren Finger um "nein" auszudrücken; nicken Sie mit dem Kopf oder heben Sie zwei Finger um "ja" auszudrücken.

(Phonetic)

Ha-loh! Ich möhh'tuh ee'nuhn hel'fuhn. Ich shpre'huh kīn doitsh, ah'buhr ich ver'duh dee'zuhs bookh bā-nüt'zuhn um zee ī'ni-guhs tsoo frah'guhn. Ich ver'duh ee'ruh ant'vor-tuhn nihht fer-shtay'uhn. Dās-halb' ant'vor-tuhn zee meer in-dām' zee ee'ruhn kopf shü'tln ō'der hāb'uhn zee ee'ruhn fing'uhr um nīn ows'tsoo-drük-uhn; nick'uhn zee mit dām kopf ō'der hāb'uhn zee tsvī fing'uhr um ya ows'tsoo-drük-uhn.

The Interpreter in Five Languages

GENERAL

Basic Questions and Replies

English	Spanish	Italian	French	German
Good morning.	Buenos días.	Buon giorno.	Bonjour.	Guten Morgen.
What is your name?	¿Cómo se llama?	Come si chiama Lei?	Quel est votre nom?	Wie heissen Sie?
How old are you?	¿Cuántos años tiene?	Quanti anni ha?	Quel âge avez-vous?	Wie alt sind Sie?
Do you understand me?	¿Me entiende?	Mi capisce?	Me comprenez-vous?	Verstehen Sie mich?
Answer only . . .	Conteste solamente . . .	Risponda solamente . . .	Répondez seulement . . .	Antworten Sie nur . . .
Yes No	Sí No	Sì No	Oui Non	Ja Nein
What do you say?	¿Qué dice?	Cosa dice?	Que dites-vous?	Was sagen Sie?
Speak slower.	Hable más despacio.	Parli più adaggio.	Parlez plus lentement.	Sprechen Sie langsamer.
Say it once again.	Repítalo, por favor.	Lo dica ancora una volta.	Répétez ça.	Wiederholen Sie das.
Don't be afraid.	No tenga miedo.	Non abbia paura.	N'ayez pas peur.	Haben Sie keine Angst.
Try to recollect.	Trate de recordar.	Cerchi di ricordarsi.	Cherchez à vous en rappeler.	Versuchen Sie sich zu erinnern.
You cannot remember?	¿No recuerda?	Non si ricorda?	Ne vous en souvenez pas?	Können Sie sich nicht erinnern?
Come to my office.	Venga a mi oficina.	Venga al mio ufficio.	Venez à mon bureau.	Kommen Sie in mein sprechzimmer
Please remove all your clothes.	Por favor, desvístase completamente.	Per cortesia, si spogli.	Veuillez-vous déshabiller.	Ziehen Sie sich bitte ganz aus.
You will?	¿Ud. quiere?*	Desidera?	Vous voulez bien?	Sie wollen?
You will not?	¿No quiere Ud.?	Non desidera?	Vous ne voulez pas?	Sie wollen nicht?
You don't know?	¿No sabe?	Non sa?	Vous ne savez pas?	Wissen Sie nicht?

* Ud.—Usted.

The Interpreter in Five Languages (Continued)

English	Spanish	Italian	French	German
Is it impossible?	¿Es imposible?	È impossibile?	C'est impossible?	Ist es unmöglich?
It is necessary.	Es necesario.	È necessario.	C'est necéssaire.	Es ist unbedingt nötig.
That is right.	Está bien.	Va bene.	C'est bien.	Das ist richtig.
Show me . . .	Enséñeme . . .	Mi faccia vedere . . .	Montrez-moi . . .	Zeigen Sie mir . . .
Here There	Aquí Allí	Qui Qua	Ici Là	Hier Da
Which side?	¿En qué lado?	Quale lato?	Quel côté?	Auf welcher Seite?
Since when?	¿Desde cuándo?	Da quando?	Depuis quand?	Seit wann?
Right	Derecha	A destra	A droit	Rechts
Left	Izquierda	A sinistra	A gauche	Links
More or less	Más o menos	Più o meno	Plus ou moins	Mehr oder weniger
How long?	¿Cuánto tiempo?	Da quanto tempo?	Combien de temps?	Wie lange?
Not much	No mucho	Non molto	Pas beaucoup	Nicht viel
Try again.	Trate otra vez.	Provi di nuovo.	Essayez encore une fois.	Versuchen Sie es noch ein mal.
Never	Nunca	Mai	Jamais	Niemals
Never mind.	Olvídelo.	Non importa.	Ça ne fait rien.	Lassen Sie es gut sein.
That will do.	Suficiente.	Basta così.	Ça suffit.	Das ist genug.
About how much daily?	¿Más o menos qué cantidad diaramente?	Circa quanto al giorno?	A peu près combien par jour?	Ungefähr wie viel täglich?
So much?	¿Tanto?	Tanto?	Autant?	So viel?
You must be very careful.	Tiene que tener mucho cuidado.	Deve usare molte precauzioni.	Vous devez prendre garde.	Sie müssen sehr vorsichtig sein.

Seasons

English	Spanish	Italian	French	German
In the spring.	En la primavera.	Nella primavera.	Au printemps.	Im Frühjahr.

English	Spanish	Italian	French	German
In summer.	En el verano.	Nell' estate.	En été.	Im Sommer.
In autumn.	En el otoño.	Nell' autunno.	En automne.	Im Herbst.
In winter.	En el invierno.	Nell' inverno.	En hiver.	Im Winter.

Months

English	Spanish	Italian	French	German
The months	Los meses	I mesi	Les mois	Die Monate
January	enero	gennaio	janvier	Januar
February	febrero	febbraio	février	Februar
March	marzo	marzo	mars	März
April	abril	aprile	avril	April
May	mayo	maggio	mai	Mai
June	junio	giugno	juin	Juni
July	julio	luglio	juillet	Juli
August	agosto	agosto	août	August
September	septiembre	settembre	septembre	September
October	octubre	ottobre	octobre	Oktober
November	noviembre	novembre	novembre	November
December	diciembre	dicembre	décembre	Dezember

Days of the Week

English	Spanish	Italian	French	German
Sunday	domingo	domenica	dimanche	Sonntag
Monday	lunes	lunedì	lundi	Montag
Tuesday	martes	martedì	mardi	Dienstag
Wednesday	miércoles	mercoledì	mercredi	Mittwoch
Thursday	jueves	giovedì	jeudi	Donnerstag
Friday	viernes	venerdì	vendredi	Freitag
Saturday	sábado	sabato	samedi	Sonnabend

The Interpreter in Five Languages (Continued)

Numbers and Time of Day
(office hours, age, diagnosis, treatment)

English	Spanish	Italian	French	German
One	Uno	Uno	Un	Eins
Two	Dos	Due	Deux	Zwei
Three	Tres	Tre	Trois	Drei
Four	Cuatro	Quattro	Quatre	Vier
Five	Cinco	Cinque	Cinq	Fünf
Six	Seis	Sei	Six	Sechs
Seven	Siete	Sette	Sept	Sieben
Eight	Ocho	Otto	Huit	Acht
Nine	Nueve	Nove	Neuf	Neun
Ten	Diez	Dieci	Dix	Zehn
Twenty	Veinte	Venti	Vingt	Zwanzig
Thirty	Treinta	Trenta	Trente	Dreissig
Forty	Cuarenta	Quaranta	Quarante	Vierzig
Fifty	Cincuenta	Cinquanta	Cinquante	Fünfzig
Sixty	Sesenta	Sessanta	Soixante	Sechzig
Seventy	Setenta	Settanta	Soixante-dix	Siebzig
At 10:00	A las diez	Alle dieci	A dix heures	Um zehn Uhr
At 2:30	A las dos y media	Alle due e mezzo	A deux heures et demie	Um halb drei
Early in the morning	Temprano por la mañana	Di buon mattino	De bon matin	Frühmorgens
In the daytime	En el día	Durante il giorno	Pendant la journée	Bei Tag
At noon	A mediodía	A mezzo giorno	A midi	Mittags
At bedtime	Al acostarse	All' ora di coricarsi	A l'heure de se coucher	Vor dem Schlafengehen
At night	Por la noche	Alla sera	Le soir	Abends

English	Spanish	Italian	French	German
Before meals	Antes de las comidas	Prima del pasto	Avant les repas	Vor den Mahlzeiten
After meals	Después de las comidas	Dopo il pasto	Après les repas	Nach den Mahlzeiten
Today	Hoy	Oggi	Aujourd'hui	Heute
Tomorrow	Mañana	Domani	Demain	Morgen
Every day	Todos los días	Ogni giorno	Chaque jour	Jeden Tag
Every hour	Cada hora	Ogni ora	Chaque heure	Jede Stunde
How long have you felt this way?	¿Desde cuándo se siente así?	Da quanto tempo si sente così?	Depuis quand vous sentez-vous comme ça?	Seit wann fühlen Sie sich so?
It came all of a sudden?	¿Vino de repente?	Venne tutto ad un tratto?	Ça vous est arrivé tout à coup?	Ist es ganz plötzlich gekommen?
For how many days or weeks?	¿Cuántos días o semanas?	Da quanti giorni o settimane?	Depuis combien de jours ou semaines?	Seit wievielen Tagen oder Wochen?
Do they come every day?	¿Los tiene todos los días?	Le vengono tutti i giorni?	Ça vous gêne tous le jours?	Kommt es jeden Tag?
At the same hour?	¿A la misma hora?	Alla stessa ora?	A la même heure?	Zur selben Stunde?
At intervals?	¿De vez en cuando?	Ad intervalli?	De temps à autre?	Dann und wann?
It will be too late.	Será demasiado tarde.	Sarà troppo tardi.	Ce sera trop tard.	Es wird zu spät sein.

Colors

English	Spanish	Italian	French	German
Black	Negro	Nero	Noir	Schwarz
Blue	Azul	Blu	Bleu	Blau
Green	Verde	Verde	Vert	Grün
Pink	Rosado	Rosa	Rose	Rosa
Red	Rojo	Rosso	Rouge	Rot
White	Blanco	Bianco	Blanc	Weiss
Yellow	Amarillo	Giallo	Jaune	Gelb

Parts of Body

English	Spanish	Italian	French	German
In the abdomen?	¿En el vientre?	Nel ventre?	Dans le abdomen?	Im Leib?

The Interpreter in Five Languages (Continued)

English	Spanish	Italian	French	German
The ankle	El tobillo	La caviglia	La cheville	**Das Fussgelenk**
The arm	El brazo	Il braccio	Le bras	Der Arm
The back	La espalda	Il dorso	Le dos	Der Rücken
The bones	Los huesos	La ossa	Le os	Die Knochen
The chest	El pecho	Il petto	La poitrine	Die Brust
The ears	Los oídos	Le orecchie	Les oreilles	Die Ohren
The elbow	El codo	Il gomito	Le coude	Der Ellenbogen
The eye	El ojo	L'occhio	L'oeil	Das Auge
The foot	**El pie**	Il piede	Le pied	Der Fuss
The gums	**Las encias**	Le gengive	**Les gengives**	**Das Zahnfleisch**
The hand	La mano	La mano	La main	Die Hand
The head	La cabeza	La testa	La tête	Der Kopf
The heart	El corazón	Il cuore	Le coeur	Das Herz
The leg	La pierna	La gamba	La jambe	Das Bein
The liver	El hígado	Il fegato	Le foie	Die Leber
The lungs	Los pulmones	I polmoni	Les poumons	Die Lungen
The mouth	La boca	La bocca	La bouche	Der Mund
The muscles	**Los músculos**	I muscoli	Les muscles	Die Muskeln
The neck	El cuello	Il collo	Le cou	Der Nacken
The nerves	Los nervios	I nervi	Les nerfs	Die Nerven
The nose	La nariz	Il naso	Le nez	Die Nase
The ribs	Las costillas	Le costole	Les côtes	Die Rippen
The shoulder blades	Las paletillas	**Le scapole**	Les omoplates	Die Schulterblatter
The side	El flanco	Il fianco	Le côté	Die Seite
The skin	La piel	La pelle	La peau	Die Haut

294

English	Spanish	Italian	French	German
The skull	El cráneo	Il cranio	Le crâne	Der Schädel
The stomach	El estómago	Lo stomaco	L'estomac	Der Magen
The teeth	Los dientes	I denti	Les dents	Die Zähne
The temples	Las sienes	Le tempie	Les tempes	Die Schläfen
The thigh	El muslo	La coscia	La cuisse	Der Oberschenkel
The throat	La garganta	La gola	La gorge	Der Hals
The thumb	El dedo pulgar	Il pollice	Le pouce	Der Daumen
The tongue	La lengua	La lingua	La langue	Die Zunge
The wrist	La muñeca	Il polso	Le poignet	Das Handgelenk

Work History

English	Spanish	Italian	French	German
What work do you do?	¿Cuál es su ocupación?	Che lavoro fa?	Quelle est votre profession?	Was ist Ihr Beruf?
Is it heavy physical work?	¿Es un trabajo corporal pesado?	È un pesante lavoro manuale?	Est-ce que c'est un travail physiquement fatigant?	Ist es eine schwere körperliche Arbeit?
What work have you done?	¿Qué trabajo ha hecho?	Che lavoro ha fatto?	A quoi avez-vous travaillé?	Welche Arbeit haben Sie getan?

HISTORY
Family

English	Spanish	Italian	French	German
Are you married?	¿Es Ud. casado?	È sposato?	Etes-vous marié?	Sind Sie verheiratet?
A widower?	¿Viudo?	È vedovo?	Veuf?	Ein Witwer?
A widow?	¿Viuda?	È vedova?	Veuve?	Eine Witwe?
Do you have children?	¿Tiene Ud. hijos?	Ha bambini?	Avez-vous des enfants?	Haben Sie Kinder?
Are they still living?	¿Viven todavía?	Vivono ancora?	Sont-ils encore vivants?	Leben sie noch?
Do you have any sisters?	¿Tiene hermanas?	Ha sorelle?	Avez-vous des soeurs?	Haben Sie Schwestern?
Do you have any brothers?	¿Tiene hermanos?	Ha fratelli?	Avez-vous des frères?	Haben Sie Brüder?
Of what did your mother die?	¿De qué murió su madre?	Di checosa è morta Sua mamma?	De quoi est morte votre mère?	Woran ist Ihre Mutter gestorben?

The Interpreter in Five Languages (Continued)

English	Spanish	Italian	French	German
And your father?	¿Y su padre?	E Suo padre?	Et votre père?	Und Ihr Vater?
Your grandfather?	¿Su abuelo?	Suo nonno?	Votre grand-père?	Ihr Grossvater?
Your grandmother?	¿Su abuela?	Sua nonna?	Votre grand-mère?	Ihre Grossmutter?

General

English	Spanish	Italian	French	German
Do you have . . . ?	¿Tiene . . . ?	Ha Lei	Avez-vous . . . ?	Haben Sie . . . ?
Have you ever had . . . ?	¿Ha tenido . . . ?	Ha mai avuto . . . ?	Avez-vous jamais eu . . . ?	Haben Sie je . . . gehabt?
Chills	Escalofríos	I brividi	Les frissons	Ein Fieberfrösteln
An attack of fever	Un ataque de calentura	Un attacco di febbre	Une attaque de fièvre	Ein Fieberanfall
Toothache	Dolor de muelas	Mal di denti	Le mal aux dents	Zahnschmerzen
Hemorrhage	Hemorragia	Emorragia	De hémorragie	Die Blutergüsse
Nosebleeds	Hemorragia por la nariz	Emorragia nasale	Saignements de nez	Das Nasenbluten
Unusual vaginal bleeding	Hemorragia vaginal fuera de los periodos	Perdite di sangue irregulari dalla vagina	Du saignement vaginal anormal	Jemals unregelmässiges bluten aus der Scheide
When did you last have a period?	¿Cuándo tuvo Ud. su última menstruación?	Quando ha avuto l'ultima volta le menstruazione?	Quand avez-vous eu vos règles pour la dernière fois?	Wann war die letze Menstruation?
Do you take birth control pills?	¿Toma Ud. píldoras anticonceptvas	Prende pillole contro la gravibanza	Est-ce que vous prenez des médicaments anti-conceptionnels?	Nehmen Sie Geburtskontroll-pillen?
Hoarseness	Ronquera	Raucedine	Enrouement	Heiserkeit

Diseases

English	Spanish	Italian	French	German
What diseases have you had?	¿Qué enfermedades ha tenido?	Che malattie ha avuto?	Quelles maladies avez-vous eues?	Welche Krankheiten haben Sie gehabt?
Allergy	Alergia	Allergie	Une maladie allergique	Überempfindlichkeiten

English	Spanish	Italian	French	German
Anemia	Anemia	Anemia	L'anémie	Blutarmut
Bleeding tendency	Tendencia a sangrar	Tendenza alle emorragie	Une tendance à saigner	Neigung zum Bluten
Cancer	Cáncer	Cancro	Le cancer	Krebs
Chicken pox	Varicela	Varicella	La varicelle	Windpocken
Diabetes	Diabetes	Diabete	Le diabète	Zuckerkrankheit
Diphtheria	Difteria	Difterite	La diphthérie	Diphtherie
German measles	Rubéola	Rosolia	Rubéole	Röteln
Gonorrhea	Gonorrea	Gonorrea	La gonorrhée	Gonorrhöe, Tripper
Heart disease	Enfermedad del corazón	Malattia di cuore	Une maladie de coeur	Herzkrankheit
High blood pressure	Presion sanguinea elevada	Pressione alta del sangue	La tension artérielle trop élevée	Hohen Blutdruck
Influenza	Gripe (influenza)	Influenza	La grippe	Grippe
Lead poisoning	Envenenamiento con plomo	Avvelenamento da piombo	Empoisonnement causé par le plomb	Bleivergiftung
Liver disease	Enfermedad del hígado	Una malattia del fegato	Une maladie de foie	Eine Leberkrankheit
Malaria	Malaria (paludismo)	Malaria	La malaria	Malaria
Measles	Sarampión	Morbillo	La rougeole	Die Masern
Mental disease	Enfermedades mentales	Malattie mentali	Une maladie mentale	Geisteskrankheit
Mumps	Paperas	Orecchioni	Les oreillons	Mumps
Nervous disease	Enfermedades nerviosas	Malattie nervose	Une maladie nerveuse	Nervenkrankheit
Pleurisy	Pleuresia	Pleurite	Une pleurésie	Rippenfellentzündung
Pneumonia	Pulmonia	Polmonite	Pneumonie	Die Lungenentzündung
Rheumatic fever	Reumatismo (fiebre reumática)	Febbre reumatica	La fièvre rhumatismale	Rheumatisches Fieber
Rheumatism	Reumatismo	Reumatismo	Le rhumatisme	Der Rheumatismus
Scarlet fever	Escarlatina	Febbre scarlattina	La fièvre scarlatine	Das Scharlachfieber
Smallpox	Viruela	Vaiolo	La variole	Pocken
Syphilis	Sífilis	Sifilide (lue)	La syphilis	Syphilis

The Interpreter in Five Languages (Continued)

English	Spanish	Italian	French	German
Tuberculosis	Tuberculosis	Tubercolosi	Tuberculose	Die Tuberkulose
Typhoid fever	Tifoidea	Febre il tifo	La fièvre typhoïde	Der Typhus

EXAMINATION
General

English	Spanish	Italian	French	German
How do you feel?	¿Cómo se siente?	Come stá?	Comment vous sentez-vous?	Wie fühlen Sie sich?
Good	Bien	Bene	Bien	Gut
Bad	Mal	Male	Mal	Schlecht
Let me see …	Déjeme ver …	Mi lasci vedere …	Permettez-moi de voir …	Lassen Sie mich sehen …
Let me feel your pulse.	Déjeme tomarle el pulso.	Mi lasci sentire il polso.	Permettez-moi de vous tâter le pouls.	Lassen Sie mich Ihren Puls fühlen.
Whisper: one, two, three.	Repita en voz baja: uno, dos, tres.	Dica piano: uno, due, tre.	Dites tout bas: un, deux, trois.	Flüstern Sie: eins, zwei, drei.
Say it out loud.	Dígalo en voz alta.	Lo dica ad alta voce.	Dites-le à voix haute.	Sagen Sie es laut.
Sit down.	Siéntese.	Si sieda.	Asseyez-vous.	Setzen Sie sich.
Stand up.	Levántese.	Si alzi.	Levez-vous.	Stehen Sie auf.
Can you not rise quicker?	¿No puede levantarse más rápidamente?	Non si può alzare un po' più presto?	Vous ne pouvez pas vous lever plus vite?	Können Sie sich nicht schneller erheben?
Walk a little way.	Ande algunos pasos.	Cammini un po'.	Faites quelques pas.	Gehen Sie einige Schritte.
Return; go backwards.	Vuelva; ande para atrás.	Ritorni; cammini all' indietro.	Revenez; allez à retours.	Kommen Sie zurück; gehen Sie rückwarts.
Do you feel like falling?	¿Le parece que se va a caer?	Si sente come se dovesse cadere?	Vous sentez vous comme si vous allez tomber?	Ist es Ihnen als ob Sie fallen werden?
Do you feel dizzy?	¿Tiene Ud. vértigo?	Ha delle vertigini?	Avez-vous le vertige?	Ist Ihnen schwindlig?
Are you tired?	¿Está Ud. cansado?	Si sente molto stanco?	Êtes vous fatigué?	Sind Sie müde?

English	Spanish	Italian	French	German
Have you slept well?	¿Ha dormido bien?	Ha dormito bene?	Avez-vous bien dormi?	Haben Sie gut geschlafen?
Have you any difficulty in breathing?	¿Tiene dificultad al respirar?	Ha difficoltà di respirare?	C'est difficile à respirer?	Fällt Ihnen das Atemholen schwer?
Have you lost weight?	¿Ha perdido Ud. peso?	È dimagrito?	Avez-vous maigri?	Haben Sie abgenommen?
Since when have you had this eruption?	¿Desde cuándo tiene esta erupción?	Da quanto ha questa eruzione?	Depuis quand avez-vous cette éruption?	Seit wann haben Sie diesen Ausschlag?
Do you sweat much at night?	¿Suda mucho por la noche?	Suda molto alla notte?	Transpirez-vous beaucoup pendant la nuit?	Schwitzen Sie viel in der Nacht?
Are you warm?	¿Tiene calor?	Ha caldo?	Avez-vous chaud?	Ist Ihnen heiss?
Are you cold?	¿Tiene frío?	Ha freddo?	Avez-vous froid?	Ist Ihnen kalt?
Have you been exposed much to the wet weather?	¿Ha estado expuesto a la intemperie?	Si è mai esposto all' umidità?	Avez-vous été longtemp sous la pluie?	Sind Sie dem feuchten Wetter ausgesetzt gewesen?
Can you eat?	¿Puede comer?	Può mangiare?	Pouvez-vous manger?	Können Sie essen?
Have you a good appetite?	¿Tiene Ud. buen apetito?	Ha buon appetito?	Avez-vous un bon appétit?	Haben Sie guten Appetit?
Are you thirsty?	¿Tiene sed?	Ha sete?	Avez-vous soif?	Haben Sie Durst?
Do you still feel very weak?	¿Se siente muy débil todavía?	Si sente ancora molto débole?	Vous sentez-vous encore très faible?	Fühlen Sie sich noch sehr schwach?
Had you been drinking?	¿Había tomado alguna bebida alcohólica?	Ha bevuto?	Est-ce que vous-aviez bu quelque chose d'alcoolique?	Waren Sie angetrunken?
Are you a drinking man?	¿Toma Ud. bebidas alcohólicas habitualmente?	Ha l'abitudine di bere?	Buvez-vous des choses alcooliques d'habitude?	Sind Sie em Trinker?
Are you nervous?	¿Está Ud. nervioso?	È nervoso?	Etes-vous nerveux?	Sind Sie nervös?
When were you first taken sick?	¿Cuándo le empezó esta enfermedad?	Quando si è ammalato la prima volta?	Quand êtes-vous tombé malade d'abord?	Wann hat diese Krankheit begonnen?
How did this illness begin?	¿Cómo empezó esta enfermedad?	Come ha incominciato questa malattia?	Comment cette maladie a-t-elle commencé?	Wie hat diese Krankheit begonnen?
Did you take anything for it?	¿Tomó algo para mejorarla?	Ha preso qual cosa per curarsi?	Avez-vous pris quelque chose pour cela?	Haben Sie etwas dafür genommen?

The Interpreter in Five Languages (Continued)

English	Spanish	Italian	French	German
Have you taken the medicine?	¿Ha tomado Ud. la medicina?	Ha preso la medicina?	Avez-vous pris la medicament?	Haben Sie die Medizin genommen?
A wound	Una herida	Una piaga	Une plaie	Eine Wunde
Are you subject to them?	¿Lo suede a menudo?	Ne è soggetto?	Ça vous gêne souvent?	Haben Sie dieselben häufig?
Did a dog bite you?	¿Lo mordió un perro?	L'ha morsicato un cane?	Est-ce qu'un chien vous a mordu?	Hat Sie eine Hund gebissen?
Did a fly sting you?	¿Lo picó una mosca?	L'ha punto una mosca?	Est-ce qu'une mouche vous a piqué?	Hat Sie eine Fliege gestochen?
Did you prick yourself with a pin?	¿Se ha pinchado con un alfiler?	Si è punto con una spilla?	Vous êtes-vous piqué avec une épingle?	Haben Sie sich mit einer Stecknadel gestochen?
Did you burn yourself?	¿Se quemó?	Si è bruciato?	Vous êtes-vous brulé?	Haben Sie sich verbrannt?
Did you sprain your foot?	¿Se torció el pie?	Si ha dislocato un piede?	Vous êtes-vous fait une entorse au pied?	Haben Sie Ihren Fuss verstaucht?

Pain

English	Spanish	Italian	French	German
Have you any pain?	¿Tiene dolor?	Ha dolori?	Avez-vous mal quelque?	Haben Sie Schmerzen?
Where does it hurt?	¿Dónde le duele?	Dove le duele?	Où avez-vous mal?	Wo haben Sie Schmerzen?
Do you have pain here?	¿Le duele aquí?	Ha dolori qui?	Avez-vous mal par ici?	Haben Sie Schmerzen hier?
Do you have a pain in your side?	¿Le duele el costado?	Avete dolori al fianco?	Avez-vous mal au côté?	Haben Sie Seitenstechen?
Show me where.	Enséñeme dónde.	Mi mostri dove.	Montrez-moi oů.	Zeigen Sie mir wo.
What did you feel in the beginning?	¿Qué sentía cuando empezó?	Che sentiva al principio?	Qu'avez-vous senti au commencement?	Was haben Sie anfangs gespürt?
Shooting pains?	¿Dolores agudos?	Dei dolori acuti?	Des elancements?	Stechende Schmerzen?
As if one were pricking you with pins?	¿Como si estuvieran pinchándole con alfileres?	Come se fossero delle spille?	Comme si l'on vous piquäit avec des épingles?	Als ob man Sie mit Stecknadeln stäche?
Did you feel much pain at the time?	¿Sintió mucho dolor entonces?	Avete sentito molto dolore allora?	Est-ce que ça vous a fait beaucoup de mal alors?	Haben Sie gleich damals arge Schmerzen gespürt?

English	Spanish	Italian	French	German
Is it worse now?	¿Está peor ahora?	È peggio ora?	Est-ce que c'est encore pire maintenant?	Ist es jetzt schlimmer?
Does it still pain you?	¿Le duele todavía?	Fa male ancora?	Est-ce que ça vous fait mal toujours?	Schmerzt er noch?
Do you still have that heavy pain?	¿Le duele mucho todavía?	Ha ancora quel dolore pesante?	Avez-vous toujours la douleur pesante?	Haben Sie noch den drückenden Schmerz?
Does it pain you to breathe?	¿Le duele al respirar?	Le fa male respirare?	Votre respiration est-elle douloureuse?	Spüren Sie Schmerzen beim Atmen?

Head

English	Spanish	Italian	French	German
How does your head feel?	¿Cómo siente la cabeza?	Come si sente la testa?	Comment va votre tête?	Wie geht es Ihrem Kopf?
Your memory	Su memoria	La sua memoria	Votre mémoire	Ihr Gedächtnis
Is it good?	¿Es buena?	È buona?	Est-elle bonne?	Ist es gut?
Have you any pain in the head?	¿Le duele la cabeza?	Ha dolor di testa?	Avez-vous mal à la tête?	Haben Sie Kopfschmerzen?
Did you fall and how did you fall?	¿Se cayó, y cómo se cayó?	È caduto, e come è caduto?	Etes-vous tombé et comment êtes-vous tombé?	Sind Sie gefallen und wie sind Sie gefallen?
Did you faint?	¿Se desmayó?	È svenuto?	Vous êtes-vous évanoui?	Sind Sie ohnmächtig geworden?
Have you ever had fainting spells?	¿Ha tenido desmayos alguna vez?	È mai svenuto regolarmente?	Avez-vous jamais eu des évanouissements?	Haben Sie jemals Ohnmachtsanfälle gehabt?

Ears

English	Spanish	Italian	French	German
Do you have ringing in the ears?	¿Le pitan los oídos?	Le tentennano le orecchie?	Avez-vous des bourdonnements d'oreilles?	Haben Sie Ohrenbrausen?
Do you have discharge from the ears?	¿Le supuran los oídos?	Le esce materia dalle orecchie?	Est-ce que vous avez un écoulement des oreilles?	Eitern Ihre Ohren?
The hearing	El oído	L'udito	L'ouïe	Das Gehör
Is it affected?	¿Está afectado?	È compromesso?	Est-elle changée?	Ist es angegriffen?

The Interpreter in Five Languages (Continued)

Eyes

English	Spanish	Italian	French	German
Look up.	Mire para arriba.	Guardi sù.	Regardez en haut.	Schauen Sie hinauf.
Look down.	Mire para abajo.	Guardi giu.	Regardez en bas.	Schauen Sie hinunter.
Look toward your nose.	Mire la nariz.	Si guardi il naso.	Regardez le nez.	Schauen Sie auf Ihre Nase.
Look at me.	Míreme.	Mi guardi.	Regardez-moi.	Sehen Sie mich an.
Can you see what is on the wall?	¿Puede ver lo que está en la pared?	Può vedere cosa c'è sui muro?	Pouvez-vous voir ce qu'il y a contre le mur?	Können Sie sehen was hier an der Wand ist?
You cannot?	¿No puede?	Non può?	Vous ne pouvez pas?	Können Sie es nicht **erkennen?**
Can you see it now?	¿Puede verlo ahora?	Può vederlo adesso?	Le voyez-vous maintenant?	Können Sie es jetzt sehen?
And now?	¿Y ahora?	Ed ora?	Et maintenant?	Und nun?
What is it?	¿Qué es ésto?	Che cosa è?	Qu'est-ce que c'est?	Was ist es?
Tell me what number it is.	Dígame qué número es éste.	Mi dica che numero è.	Dites-moi quel est le numéro.	Sagen Sie mir welche Nummer es ist.
Tell me what letter it is.	Dígame qué letra es ésta.	Mi dica che lettera è.	Dites-moi quelle est la lettre.	Nennen Sir mir diesen Buchstaben.
Do you see things through a mist?	¿Ve las cosas a través de una niebla?	Vede le cose come se fossero fra la nebbia?	Voyez-vous les choses à travers d'un brouillard?	Sehen Sie alles durch einen Nebel?
Can you see clearly?	¿Puede ver claramente?	Può vedere chiaro?	Pouvez-vous voir clairement?	Sehen Sie **deutlich?**
Better at a distance?	¿Mejor a cierta distancia?	Meglio a distanza?	Mieux à distance?	Besser aus **der Entfernung?**
Do your eyes water a good deal?	¿Le lagrimean mucho los ojos?	Le lacrimano molto gli occhi?	Est-ce que les yeux vous coulent beaucoup?	Tränen Ihre Augen stark?
Can't you open your eye?	¿No puede abrir el ojo?	Non puo aprire l'occhio?	Ne pouvez-vous pas ouvrir l'oeil?	Können Sie Ihr Auge nicht öffnen?
Do not try to open it when you awaken.	No trate de abrirlo al despertarse.	Quando si sveglia si forzi ad aprirlo.	N'essayez pas de l'ouvrir en vous réveillent.	Versuchen Sie nicht, es beim Aufwachen zu öffnen.

English	Spanish	Italian	French	German
Did anything get into your eye?	¿Le entró algo en el ojo?	Le è entrata qualche cosa nell'occhio?	Est-ce que quelque chose est entré dans l'oeil?	Ist Ihnen etwas ins Auge geflogen?
Do you sometimes see things double?	¿Ve las cosas doble algunas veces.	Vede qualche volta le cose doppie?	Est-ce que la vue est **double parfois?**	Sehen Sie manchmal doppelt?
Does the eyeball feel as if it were swollen?	¿Le parece que el ojo está hinchado?	Le sembra che l'occhio sia gonfio?	L'oeil vous semble-t-il gonflé?	Fühlt sich das Auge wie **geschwollan?**
You must be careful not to go out yet.	Tenga cuidado de no salir todavía.	Deve aver cura a non andar fuori.	Gardez de sortir maintenant.	Sie dürfen durchaus noch nicht ausgehen.
It would harm your eyes.	Le haría daño a los ojos.	Le farà male agli occhi.	Cela vous abîmerait les yeux.	Es würde Ihren Augen schaden.
Since when has your eyesight failed you?	¿Desde cuándo ha disminuido su vista?	Da quanto tempo la sua **vista È diminuita?**	Depuis quand votre vue s'est-elle diminuée?	Seit wann hat Ihre Sehkraft nachgelassen?

Throat and Mouth

English	Spanish	Italian	French	German
Cough.	Tosa.	Tossisca.	Toussez.	Husten Sie.
Cough again.	Tosa otra vez.	Tossisca ancora.	Toussez encore une fois.	Husten Sie noch einmal.
Open your mouth.	Abra la boca.	Apra la bocca.	Ouvrez la bouche.	Öffnen Sie den Mund.
Does it hurt you to open your mouth?	¿Le duele al abrir la boca?	Le fa male aprir la bocca?	Ouvrir la bouche vous fait-il mal?	Spüren Sie Schmerzen wenn Sie den Mund öffnen?
Since when do you cough?	¿Desde cuándo tose Ud?	Da quando ha la tosse?	Depuis quand avez-vous la toux?	Seit wann husten Sie?
You cough a little?	¿Tose poco?	Tossisca poco?	Toussez-vous un peu?	Husten Sie manchmal?
Take a deep breath.	Respire profundamente.	Prenda un gran respiro.	Respirez profondément.	Atmen Sie tief.
Do you expectorate much?	¿Escupe mucho?	Sputa molto?	Crachez-vous beaucoup?	Spucken Sie viel aus?
What is the color of your expectorations?	¿De qué color es el esputo?	Di che color lo sputo?	De quelle sont vos crachats?	Welche Farbe hat der Speichel?
Does your tongue feel swollen?	¿Siente Ud. la lengua hinchada?	Ha la lingua gonfia?	Est-ce que la langue vous paraît gonflée?	Fühlt sich Ihre Zunge wie **geschwollenan?**
Do you have a sore throat?	¿Le duele la garganta?	Ha mal di gola?	Avez-vous mal à la gorge?	Haben Sie **Halsschmerzen?**
Does it hurt to swallow?	¿Le duele al tragar?	Quando ingoia le fa male?	Ça vous fait mal à avaler?	Spüren Sie Schmerzen beim Schlucken?

303

The Interpreter in Five Languages (*Continued*)

English	Spanish	Italian	French	German
Arms and Hands				
Let me see your hand.	Enséñeme la mano.	Mi faccia vedere la sua mano.	Montrez-moi la main.	Zeigen Sie mir Ihre Hand.
Have you no power in it?	¿No tiene fuerza en la mano?	Non ha forza nella mano?	Est-elle complètement inerte?	Ist sie ganz kraftlos?
Grasp my hand.	Apriete mi mano.	Mi stringa la mano.	Serrez-moi la main.	Drücken Sie mir die Hand.
Can you not do it better than that?	¿No puede hacerlo más fuerte?	Non può far meglio?	Vous ne **pouvez-pas serrer plus** fort que cela?	Können Sie nicht fester greifen?
Your arm feels paralyzed?	¿Parece que el brazo está paralizado?	Si sente il braccio paralizzato?	Est-ce que le bras vous paraît paralysé?	Ihr Arm erscheint Ihnen gelähmt?
Raise your arm.	Levante el brazo.	Alzi il braccio.	Levez le bras.	Heben Sie den Arm.
Raise it more.	Más alto.	Ancora di più.	Plus haut.	Höher.
Now the other.	Ahora el otro.	Adesso l'altro.	Maintenant l'autre.	Jetzt den andern.
Since when is your arm so powerless?	Desde cuándo no tiene fuerza en el brazo?	Da quando il suo braccio è senza forza?	Depuis quand votre bras a-t-il perdu la force?	Seit wann ist Ihr Arm so kraftlos?
Had you been sleeping on your arm?	¿Ha dormido encima del brazo?	Ha dormito col braccio sotto la testa?	Vous êtes-vous endormi sur le bras?	Sind Sie auf Ihrem Arm eingeschlafen?
Gastrointestinal				
Do you have stomach cramps?	¿Tiene calambres en el estómago?	Ha dei dolori acuti allo stomaco?	Avez-vous des crampes de l'estomac?	Haben Sie Magenkrämpfe?
Since when is your tongue that color?	¿Desde cuándo tiene la lengua de ese color?	Da quando la sua lingua è di questo colore?	Depuis quand votre langue a-t-elle cette couleur?	Seit wann hat Ihre Zunge diese Farbe?
Have you a pain in the pit of your stomach?	¿Tiene dolor en la boca del estómago?	Ha dei dolori alla bocca dello stomaco?	Est-ce que ça vous fait mal dans le creux de l'estomac?	Haben Sie Schmerzen in der Magengrube?

304

Nausea	Náusea	La nausea	La nausée	Die Übelkeit
Does eating make you vomit?	¿El comer le hace vomitar?	Vomita dopo aver manginto?	Rendez-vous ce que vous mangez?	Erbrechen Sie nachdem Sie gegessen haben?
How are your stools?	¿Cómo son sus defecaciones?	Come va di corpo?	Comment allez-vous à la selle?	Wie ist der Stuhlgang?
Are they regular?	¿Son regulares?	Va regolarmente?	Allez-vous à la selle régulièrment?	Ist er regelmässig?
Have you noticed their color?	¿Se ha fijado en el color?	Si è accorto di che colore?	Avez-vous remarqué la couleur de vos selles?	Haben Sie auf die Farbe geachtet?
Are you constipated?	¿Está estreñido?	È stitico?	Etes-vous constipé?	Leiden Sie an Verstopfung?
Do you have diarrhea?	¿Tiene diarrea?	Ha diarrea?	Avez-vous la diarrhée?	Haben Sie Durchfall?
Do you pass any blood?	¿Con sangre?	Passa sangue?	Y-a-t-il du sang?	Ist Blut im Stuhl?
Have you vomited?	¿Ha vomitado?	Ha vomitato?	Avez-vous vomi?	Haben Sie erbrochen?
Do you still vomit?	¿Vomita todavía?	Vomita ancora?	Vomissez-vous encore?	Erbrechen Sie noch immer?
Do you vomit blood?	¿Vomita sangre?	Vomita sangue?	Vomissez-vous du sang?	Erbrechen Sie Blut?
Is it of a dark or bright red color?	¿Es de color rojo oscuro o claro?	È di colore rosso chiaro o rosso scuro?	La couleur du sang est elle fonçée ou claire?	Ist es dunkel oder hellrot?

Kidneys

Have you any difficulty passing water?	¿Tiene dificultad en orinar?	Ha della difficoltà nell' urinare?	Avez-vous de la difficulté à uriner?	Haben Sie Schwierigkeiten beim Wasserlassen?
Do you pass water involuntarily?	¿Orina sin querer?	Urina involontariamente?	Urinez-vous involontaire-ment?	Lassen Sie den Harn ohne es zu wollen?
Are any of your limbs swollen?	¿Están hinchados alguno de sus miembros?	Si sente gonfio in qualche parte?	Avez-vous des membres gonflés?	Ist irgendeines Ihrer Glieder geschwollen?
How long have they been swollen like this?	¿Desde cuándo están hinchados así?	Da quanto tempo che li ha cosi gonfi?	Depuis quand sont-ils gonflés comme ça?	Seit wann sind sie so angeschwollen?
Were they ever swollen before?	¿Han estado hinchados alguna vez antes?	Sono stati mai gonfi prima?	Ont-ils jamais été gonflés autrefois?	Sind sie je früher so angeschwollen gewesen?

The Interpreter in Five Languages (Continued)

TREATMENT
General

English	Spanish	Italian	French	German
It is nothing serious.	No es nada grave.	Non è nulla.	Ce n'est rien de grave.	Es ist nichts ernstliches.
You will get better.	Ud. se mejorará.	Si sentirà meglio.	Vous vous remettrez.	Es wird besser werden.
Do exactly as I tell you.	Haga exactamente lo que le digo.	Faccia estattamente ciò che Le dico.	Faites exactement ce que je vous dis.	Tun Sie genau was ich Ihnen sage.
Take a bath.	Tome un baño.	Si faccia un bagno.	Prenez un bain.	Nehmen Sie ein bad
A sponge bath	Un baño de esponja	Un bagno con la spugna	Un bain à l'éponge	Ein Schwamm bad
A bran bath	Un baño de salvado	Un bagno con crusca	Un bain au son	Ein Kleie bad
A soda bath	Un baño de soda	Un bagno con soda	Un bain à la soude	Ein Soda bad
Bathe with hot water.	Báñese con agua caliente.	Faccia il bagno con acqua calda.	Baignez-vous dans de l'eau chaude.	Baden Sie mit heissem Wasser.
Bathe with cold water.	Báñese con agua fría.	Si faccia il bagno con acqua fredda.	Baignez-vous dans de l'eau froide.	Baden Sie mit kaltem Wasser.
Bathe with alcohol.	Báñese con alcohol.	Si bagni con alcool.	Baignez-vous avec de l'alcool.	Reiben Sie sich alkoholab.
Paint the swelling with this.	Pinte la hinchazón con esto.	Deve pitturare il gonfiore con questo.	Badigeonnez l'enflure avecceci.	Pinseln Sie die Geschwulst damit.
I will use electricity.	Usaré electricidad.	Userò dell'elettricità.	Je ferai un traitment a la electricité.	Ich werde elektrischen Strom anwenden.
Apply bandage to . . .	Ponga un vendaje a . . .	Si metta una fasciatura . . .	Mettez un bandage à . . .	Verbinden Sie . . .
Apply ointment	Aplíquese ungüento.	Applichi un unguento.	Appliquez un onguent.	Verwenden Sie Salbe.
Keep very quiet.	Estése muy quieto.	Sia tranquillo.	Restez tranquille.	Verhalten Sie sich sehr ruhig.
You must not speak.	No debe hablar.	Non deve parlare.	Vous ne devez pas parler.	Sie dürfen nicht sprechen.
Swallow small pieces of ice.	Trague pedacitos de hielo.	Ingoi dei pezzettini di ghiaccio.	Avalez de petits morceaux de glace.	Schlucken Sie kleine Eisstücke.

Diet

English	Spanish	Italian	French	German
In a few days you may eat food.	Dentro de algunos días podrá comer.	Fra pochi giorni potrà mangiare.	Après quelques jours vous pouvez prendre de la nourriture.	In einigen Tagen dürfen Sie essen.
And remain on a diet.	Y estar a dieta.	E rimanga a dieta.	Et suivez un régime.	Und Diät halten.
You may eat . . .	Puede comer . . .	Potrà mangiare . . .	Vous pouvez manger . . .	Sie dürfen essen . . .
Two eggs	Dos huevos	Due d'uova	Deux oeufs	Zwei Eier
Toast	Pan tostado	Pane tostato	Du pain grillé	Geröstetes Brot
Bread	Pan	Pane	Du pain	Das Brot
Oysters	Ostras	Delle óstriche	Des huîtres	Die Austern
Chicken	Pollo	Pollo	Du poulet	Das Huhn
You may drink icewater.	Puede tomar agua con hielo.	Lei può bere acqua ghiacciata.	Vous pouvez boir de l'eau glacée.	Sie dürfen Eiswasser trinken.
Milk	Leche	Latte	Du lait	Die Milch
Tea	Té	Il té	Du thé	Der Tee
Coffee	Café	Il caffè	Du café	Der Kaffee
Chocolate	Chocolate	La cioccolatta	Du chocolat	Die Schokolade
Beef bouillon	Caldo de carne	Brodo	Le bouillon	Die Bouillon

Operation

English	Spanish	Italian	French	German
An operation will be necessary.	Tendrá que operarse.	Una operazione è necessaria.	Il faut que l'on fasse une operation.	Eine Operation ist notwendig.
We will operate . . .	Lo operaremos . . .	Opereremo . . .	Nous opérerons . . .	Wir werden operieren . . .

The Interpreter in Five Languages (*Continued*)

Medication
(use with numbers and time of day)

English	Spanish	Italian	French	German
I will give you something for that.	Le daré algo para eso.	Le darò qualche cosa per questo.	Je vous donnerai quelque chose pour cela.	Ich werde Ihnen etwas dafur geben.
I will leave a prescription.	Le dejaré una receta.	Lascerò una ricetta.	Je laisserai une ordonnance.	Ich werde Ihnen ein Rezept hierlassen.
Use it regularly.	Tómelo con regularidad.	Lo usi regolarmente.	Servez-vous-en régulièrment.	Gebrauchen Sie es regelmässig.
Take one teaspoonful three times daily (in water).	Tome una cucharadita tres veces al dia, con agua.	Ne beva un cucchiaio tre volte al giorno (con acqua).	Prenez-en une petite cuiller trois fois par jour (avec de l'eau).	Nehmen Sie einen Teelöffel voll dreimal taglich (mit Wasser).
Gargle.	Haga gárgaras.	Faccia gargarismi.	Gargarisez-vous.	Gurgeln Sie.
Use injection.	Use una inyección.	Si faccia un iniezione.	Utilises des injections.	Injizieren Sie.
Take a purgative.	Tome una purga.	Un purgante	Prenez une purgative.	Nehmen Sie ein Abführmittel.
A pill	Una píldora	Una pillola	Une pilule	Eine Pille
A powder	Un polvo	Una polverina	Une poudre	Ein Pulver
Drop into one eye.	Vierta gotas en un ojo.	Metta delle gocce nell'occhio	Faites tomber une goutte dans l'oeil.	Träufeln Sie in das eine Auge.
Drop into each eye.	Vierta gotas en cada ojo.	Metta delle gocce in ciascun occhio.	Faites tomber une goutte dans chaque oeil.	Träufeln Sie in beide Augen.

308

Index

A "t" following a page number indicates a table. An "f" following a page number indicates a figure.

318 □ Respiratory Facts